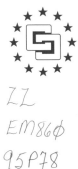

European Foundation
for the Improvement of
Living and Working Conditions

☑ **W9-CGN-078**

Public Welfare Services and Social Exclusion

**The development of
consumer-oriented initiatives
in the European Union**

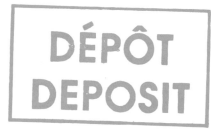
EF/95/13/EN

Nicholas Deakin started his career as a civil servant in the British Home Office and then moved on to social research, taking a doctorate at Sussex University and working on the Nuffield Foundation's survey of race relations in Britain. Subsequently he worked at the Greater London Council, as Head of Central Policy Unit and then went to Birmingham University as Professor of Social Policy and Administration. He has been an advisor to Government departments, and chaired local and national voluntary bodies. His publications include *Consuming Public Services* (with Tony Wright MP) and *The Politics of Welfare*.

Ann Davis is Director of Social Work Research and Development, The University of Birmingham. She teaches, researches and publishes in the areas of gender, health and personal social services and social work. She is actively involved as a consultant with service user groups and the staff of health and personal social services organisations.

Neil Thomas is a Senior Lecturer in the Department of Social Policy and Social Work, School of Social Science at the University of Birmingham. He directed the Department's Social Services Unit and was founding editor of *Social Services Research*. He contributed to the collection *Consuming Public Services* and wrote the essay on social services in *Learning from Innovation*, which he co-edited.

European Foundation
for the Improvement of
Living and Working Conditions

Public Welfare Services and Social Exclusion

The development of consumer-oriented initiatives in the European Union

Nicholas Deakin
Ann Davis
Neil Thomas

Loughlinstown House,
Shankill, Co. Dublin, Ireland
Tel.: (+353) 1 282 6888 Fax: (+353) 1 282 6456

Cataloguing data can be found at the end of this publication

Luxembourg: Office for Official Publications of the European Communities, 1995

ISBN 92-827-4907-X

Printed in Ireland

PREFACE

Under economic pressure to make better use of often shrinking resources in the context of growing demand, public authorities across the European Union have been rethinking and restructuring the services they fund and deliver. A considerable part of this process has been aimed at making public services more responsive to the needs and preferences of their users, i.e. consumer-oriented action.

This report forms the final synthesis of the results of a Foundation research project undertaken between 1991 and 1994 to assess these developments in a selected number of Member States (Germany, Greece, Portugal, United Kingdom, Denmark, France, Italy and Ireland). The research, which included national reviews of policies and programmes and case studies of innovative consumer-oriented initiatives, concentrated on developments in public welfare services, in particular social security and social services, which were seen to be of particular significance for disadvantaged and socially excluded persons.

The main objectives of the study, which forms an integral part of the Foundation's programme on social cohesion, were to document and assess reform and innovation in public welfare services and to consider the implications of these for service users, providers and policy makers/administrators. Additional objectives were to consider the role of women, who are disproportionately represented among users "in need" and amongst service delivery workers, especially those on the front line, and to assess the potential for further development and transfer of good practice.

The research has confirmed the central relevance of the key themes of the project, namely the persistence in the Member States of social exclusion; the wide variety of issues affecting the key actors (consumer/citizens, staff, managers and policy makers), and the lack of attention to equal opportunities and in particular to gender issues. New programmes to improve service quality and consumer orientation have consistently suffered from problems of funding and continuity. Insufficient attention has been paid to monitoring and evaluation, and thus also to transfer of successful practice.

The report analyses the strengths and weaknesses of the different approaches taken by public welfare services to improving service quality and responsiveness, and makes a series of recommendations relating to the role of users/consumers, the challenges facing staff and their trade unions, the implications for managers and policy makers, and the contribution of the European Union. These focus on the need for a greater interaction and dialogue between the key actors and systems to support this; improved training for staff and management; adequate monitoring and evaluation, paying more attention to the impacts of services on economic and social cohesion; exchange of information and experience, and greater political support, including more attention to longer term cost effectiveness and democratic accountability. It is felt that the European Union could make an important contribution in supporting positive developments, encouraging dialogue and increasing knowledge and exchange of experience.

On 26 April 1995 this report was assessed by an evaluation committee on behalf of the Foundation's Administrative Board. The participants felt that the project had given rise to very worthwhile results. The employers' representative, speaking from a private sector perspective, noted their increasing interest in the issues raised by the report. This arose in three ways - their involvement as "corporate citizens" (enterprises citoyennes), increasing privatisation of public services and as contributors to social security. He agreed with the need emphasised in the report to identify the clearly different interests of users, staff and managers in public services developments

Both trade union representatives welcomed the report and were pleased to see the emphasis on social exclusion, while stressing that not all the questions of unions in the area of public services (an issue of priority for ETUC) could be answered by this report. In their general comments they pointed to the different winners and losers in these developments, who could vary over time and location; the issue of cohesion of the public services themselves and their income and expenditure problems; the question of how to put an economic value on investments to maintain social cohesion and the need for public and private sectors to work together to combat exclusion. The relationship between consumerism and citizenship and the essential differences between private and public services were also emphasised.

The government representative said the report provided a very useful platform to highlight current EU experience and could form a good starting point for a broader discussion. It could also lead to demands for further research since the problems of reconciling resources and needs is a major problem for public services in the EU Member States.

The European Commission (DGV) felt the work of the Foundation in this area was exactly what it needed and looked forward to further collaboration on these issues in the future. Of particular concern to DGV, as elaborated in the Medium Term Social Action Programme (1995-97), was the relationship between social protection and employment. The participant from OECD gave information on its work in this area within the Public Management Service and stressed the need for more information on what is happening in public services. The impact of service quality initiatives needs much greater examination especially to identify who was benefiting and who was losing from the changes. There was also a need for greater clarity about the problem being tackled - was it about better delivery of existing services or about assessing what services are delivered in relation to needs and where were the gaps? The key role of the political process in designing and assessing programmes should also be highlighted.

Following this discussion the report was unanimously approved for publication. In relation to the conclusions and recommendations, the evaluation committee felt the report provided a good framework for the development of new ideas and actions. They stressed the need for further dialogue and networking. Improvements to public services in future would have to be seen to be cost effective and to impact on key issues such as unemployment and exclusion. There was a need for more debate, especially amongst the social partners, on how to combine public and market approaches and what is the appropriate intervention of the State to develop and maintain social cohesion. There was support expressed for more dialogue at EU level, especially by the trade union representatives, and the need to establish a European level body to represent the users' interests, especially disadvantaged users. The importance of citizens' rights and involvement was raised and the need for transparency and means for the expression of the legitimate interests of the different actors at EU level.

Wendy O'Conghaile
Robert Anderson

Research Managers

Dublin, June 1995

CONTENTS

ACKNOWLEDGEMENTS

The authors of the final report wish to acknowledge help received in its preparation from the research managers at the European Foundation, Robert Anderson and Wendy O'Conghaile and from members of the national research teams. They are also grateful for help from colleagues at the University of Birmingham, especially Helen Harris.

INTRODUCTION

Purpose of the Report

This report sets out to address one of the most significant problems that the countries of the European Union now face. The greatly increased prosperity now being experienced by the majority of the Union's citizens has not been evenly distributed. Alongside the general growth in wealth, the past decade has seen an increase in the numbers of those in poverty and a hardening of the divisions which exclude the less fortunate from access to goods and services of quality. Such divisions are present to a greater or lesser degree in all the countries of the Union and affect the same groups within them: the unemployed (especially the long-term unemployed), women, the elderly, those with disabilities and recent immigrants (EFILWC, 1994).

These divisions pose a formidable challenge for the public services of EU countries. Instead of providing a ladder for the less fortunate to climb, these services find themselves serving as a safety net. The cost of providing social protection has increased and its effectiveness has come into question - the safety net has become a spiders' web that traps those whom it purports to protect.

The contention of this report is that an effective way of addressing these problems is through reforms in the public welfare services which will make them more responsive to the requirements of consumers and especially those groups in most need. Such reforms (it will be argued) can benefit not just consumers but also the managers and staff who provide the services. They can be achieved in harmony with the goals of greater efficiency and cost effectiveness. Above all, they offer a means for promoting the social cohesion which is in danger of being lost.

Origins of the Study

The report is based primarily on research undertaken by the European Foundation for the Improvement of Living and Working Conditions. The main aims of the study, which

1

forms an integral part of the Foundation's longer term programme of work on public services, were:

- to document and assess new initiatives in public services, designed to improve quality for their users and consumers, with particular emphasis on public welfare services used by disadvantaged people;

- to consider the implications of these initiatives for service users, service providers and policy makers/administrators;

- to consider the role of women who are disproportionately represented among users "in need" and amongst service delivery workers;

- to examine the potential for development and transfer of good practice; and to contribute to policy and practice improvements at European Union and Member State level.

The study has been conducted in two phases. In the first, overviews of consumer-oriented developments in four countries (Germany, Greece, Portugal and the United Kingdom) were prepared, reviewing the changes that had taken place in each country and prospects for future developments. National overview reports were then also prepared for a second group of countries, namely Denmark, France, Ireland and Italy.

In the second phase, case studies were undertaken of two innovative consumer-oriented initiatives in each country. The case studies were selected on the following basis:

- they were drawn from the **welfare services** and concentrated in those which are of particular relevance for disadvantaged groups;

- they were related to **mainstream** services (like social services and pensions) which are used by a substantial proportion of the population, not specialised ones

2

catering for small groups; these were also services in which significant consumer-oriented initiatives had been identified in the preliminary reviews;

-   they were intended to include a wide range of **different agencies**, including central and local government, for-profit and voluntary agencies and informal and self-help groups; and

-   they were chosen to represent key dimensions of consumer-oriented change, specifically improving consumer access to services and increasing consumer influence or control over them.

The Present Report

The findings from both phases of the study are consolidated in the present report, which sets out to provide:

-   a brief overview of relevant changes currently taking place throughout the European Union;

-   an analysis of the initiatives taking place at national level in the eight countries studied; with a short discussion of issues arising from these and other attempts to promote consumer involvement in public services;

-   a summary and evaluation of the sixteen case studies undertaken and a review of the key lessons learned from them about the quality and effectiveness of the public services provided, with special emphasis on the equal opportunities dimension; and

-   key conclusions from the study overall, together with a suite of outline proposals, identifying priority areas for future action at EU and national level.

Terms Employed

Discussion of public services in the report concentrates on those that deliver welfare and a broad range of social services. Because confusion may arise, both in relation to the services themselves and the status of those that use them, we have provided a brief glossary of the terms employed (Appendix 1).

We recognise that there is currently considerable debate about the use of these terms. For example, when we refer to 'public welfare services' we include both those agencies that are responsible for the services overall and those that actually deliver them, though these may not be formally in the public sector. We should also make it clear that when we refer to 'consumers' we employ that term to describe those receiving or using public welfare services. It is sometimes assumed that to employ the word 'consumer' is to imply that there is an exact equivalence between the delivery of public services and commercial transactions between the purchasers of goods and services and their suppliers. We do not suggest that this is always or even usually so. Nevertheless, we will normally use the term 'consumer' as the closest approximation to a generally accepted and understood term in current use across the EU. However, we have retained the word 'user' in a minority of cases, where it is the preferred national usage and to change it would create unnecessary confusion.

In some other contexts, we have employed the word 'citizen'. This helps to underline the point that, in our capacity as citizens, we all share responsibility for the disadvantages that too many of our fellow inhabitants of EU countries experience and for the measures taken to address their problems.

Audience for Report

The report is designed to serve as a basis for informed discussion by policy- makers on the contribution of public services to combating social exclusion. It provides new information on strategies to strengthen this contribution and directs attention to those responsible for the development and implementation of policy - public authorities, social partners, consumers and citizens. The promotion of economic and social cohesion is now high on the European Union policy agenda and the focus of debate at all levels of decision making. There is now urgent need for further discussion of the role of public welfare services in tackling social exclusion, the implications of current changes in these services, and the action that should now be taken at all levels.

CHAPTER ONE :   The Broad Context

The European Union is passing through a period of rapid change. The turbulence associated with this change is affecting many of its citizens in a number of fundamental ways, which touch a whole range of different aspects of their lives.

Seen from one perspective, the history since the Treaty of Rome of the countries that now make up the Union has been one of remarkable success. In its present form, the Union contains only 7% of the world's working age population; yet it produces some 30% of world GDP and 45% of world trade in manufactured goods (European Commission, 1993a). Those achievements have been reflected in a rapidly rising standard of living over the past thirty years for the majority of the Union's population.

Yet alongside these successes a growing number of stresses have developed, which are affecting an increasingly large number of the population of the Union. These stresses, which had mostly been concealed by the expansion of the various national economies, have emerged into the open in different countries over the last two decades. They have taken a variety of forms, with some significant differences between regions and groups of Member States.

Causes of Stress: Unemployment

The stresses associated with the persistence of high rates of unemployment have been underlined in the recent EU White Paper on Growth, Competitiveness and Employment. The economies of the member countries of the Union have all passed through a sequence of booms and busts since the oil price shock of 1973. Improved techniques of economic management have enabled most governments to limit the adverse effects of the downswings. But with each successive recovery the basic level of unemployment has moved steadily upwards; a 'ratchet effect' is in operation, with the result that "full employment can no longer be taken for granted as the outcome of growth-creating economic policies" (European Commission 1993:17). Over the past three years, recorded unemployment has risen sharply, until it has reached 16 million people - 10.9% of the registered workforce (1994), over half of which is long-term unemployment. Although individual states have differing levels of unemployment, this is a phenomenon that affects them all.

Moreover, Europe's record in the creation of jobs has been poor; the proceeds of the benefits of growth, as it has begun to return over the past two years, have mainly been absorbed by those who have remained in employment. The European Union's employment rate - the proportion of its population of working age that is in work - is the lowest of any industrialised part of the world: less than 60% of the population, compared with 70% in Japan and the United States (European Commission 1993b). The result has been that growing numbers of the adult population are excluded from the labour force and many young people have been unable to enter it.

In part, these exclusions are due to structural changes that have taken place in the economies of the member countries and in the globalisation of the economy in general. These have affected all sectors of the economy: primary, manufacturing and service industries. The coal, shipbuilding and steel industries in the European Union have declined rapidly over this period; and other industries have also been affected by the introduction of new technologies and innovations in business practice. Some, though not all, of the resulting job losses have been made up by the development of service sector activity and new industries based on advanced technologies; but some of these are themselves now shedding labour. In any case, the new jobs created in this way have generally not gone to those areas or to those workers most affected by the decline in the older industries (EFILWC, 1994).

Alongside the advantages conferred by the completion of the Single Market, the Cecchini report (1988) referred to the importance of administering a 'supply side shock' to the economies of Europe by opening up internal markets to the effects of greater competition. It was accepted that there would be sectors of European industry that would be especially vulnerable to the consequences of this shock. For example, it was anticipated that the intensification of competition and the reduction of subsidy would have a particularly sharp impact on agricultural industries and farming - still a substantial source of employment in many European countries (Baine et al, 1992). However, the full effects of the recession that has affected all European Union countries to a greater or lesser degree over the past three years, coming as it did at this time of accelerating structural change, were not anticipated.

At the same time, most European countries have also experienced changes in the nature of work. The decline of traditional manufacturing industry means fewer assembly line jobs; the rise of services has facilitated growth in part-time and casual employment. Office work has typically become less secure, and is often undertaken on a sub-contracted or short-term basis. Technological change in advanced industries has fostered an increase in 'screwdriver' work, requiring little physical strength but much manual dexterity. Many of the new jobs being created in these ways are likely to be done by women. Other jobs in this sector have been lost to countries outside the Union, where the cost of labour is lower. The growth of low paid jobs has increased dependency on family income supports; at the same time, there is less protection for workers in these jobs.

Causes of Stress: Economic and Social Change

These economic changes have been taking place alongside a series of important social and demographic changes with which they have interacted. All European countries have experienced an ageing of their populations. It is estimated that there are now over 68 million people aged 60 or over in the European Union, representing about one fifth of the total population. By 2020 more than a quarter of the population of the present Union will have reached their sixtieth birthday (Eurostat, 1993). This has been coupled with a fall in the numbers of those who remain economically active at the end of what was previously considered to be a normal span of working life. This has produced a situation in which there are many more 'young-old' people (sometimes referred to as 'Third Age') in the non-employed populations of most European countries. The young-old, in general, are a significant consumer group and a political force likely to demand better services. At the same time, the universal rapid increase in numbers of 'old-old' people (sometimes termed 'Fourth Age': those whose physical and sometimes mental competence is beginning to fail) creates pressure for additional resources of care and support. They are especially dependent on state transfers for financial support and their social isolation presents a challenge to deliver the high quality and better co-ordinated services which can markedly improve their well-being (EFILWC, 1993).

Traditionally, key elements of this caring role have been assigned to families and to the unwaged work of women. However, changes in family structures that have affected all European countries to a greater or lesser degree suggest that while the demand for care is growing, the supply is under increasing pressure. The smaller family now faces the crises of four generations. Fewer marriages and higher divorce rates now lead to substantially more single parent households (especially in Northern Europe). More households are likely to need help from the wider network (EFILWC, 1993, op cit).

The substantial increase in the proportion of women (both married and single) who have entered the labour force interacts in complex ways with these socio-demographic trends and with policies towards the family. The character of women's work in Europe is more frequently part-time and usually insecure, sometimes undertaken at home on subcontracts and, above all, low paid. Average women's wages in Europe have been estimated as being 31% less than those of men (Baine et al, 1992: 104). Yet at the same time women have not been shielded from the effects of structural change; many of the industries in which they have traditionally worked (eg textiles) have been among those strongly affected by the globalisation of production. So there is an apparent paradox, of women experiencing simultaneously an increase in both employment and unemployment.

The nature of the work on offer and the poor financial rewards exacerbate the pressures on women who are major family wage earners. Nor does that work necessarily fit with other obligations. As the Foundation has commented in an earlier report, part-time employment has become one of the most common ways across Europe for women to combine work with family obligations. However, it is clear that not all part-time working arrangements suit the needs of women, which can have important consequences for their ability to function successfully both at work and at home (EFILWC, 1994).

The economic expansion of the Union has attracted a large number of people migrating for employment - both those moving between EU countries and those entering from outside (the estimated total black and third world population in the EU in 1992 was 15m (Baine et al, 1992). Migrants are often recruited to those industries in which indigenous workers are no longer prepared to work; and these are also often those that have been most severely affected by structural changes and by successive recessions. As a result, these groups are also experiencing higher rates of registered unemployment (eg in Holland, 35% of Turks and 42% of Moroccans are unemployed compared with 7% of 'ethnic Dutch' (Economist, 30.7.94). There are issues here of lack of skills and inadequate education, as well as endemic discrimination on racial grounds blocking access to better jobs, obstacles which are accentuated by recent outbreaks of xenophobia in some European countries and the gains made by extreme right wing political parties. There are also issues around the lack of rights of both EU and non-EU citizens, who may find themselves driven into taking work in the 'black economy'. One consequence of these forms of social exclusion is that public services will need to become more sensitive to the needs of minorities.

One of the most important results of these various changes has been the increase in poverty within the Union. If the definition of poverty employed is that of persons living in households with income of less than half the national average, there are 52m people in the European Union living in poverty (European Commission, 1994). A broader definition of 'new poverty' employed in the EU's Poverty Programme suggests that there have been increases among certain specific groups: those in marginal or insecure employment; those who had taken early retirement on reduced pensions; migrants, travellers, the homeless and women (who frequently do not appear in official unemployment statistics) and among single parents and the unemployed (Ditch, 1993).

European Union countries also have in common the failure of any increased prosperity to translate itself either into the kind of jobs needed to reduce long-term unemployment or as wealth to 'trickle down' to the poor. Loic Wacquant comments that:

"Roughly, until the 1970s, the expansion of the economy translated into improvements at the bottom of the class structure. Now when the economy goes into a downward spiral, neighbourhoods of exclusion get worse. But when it goes into an upward progression, they don't join in." (quoted in Economist, op cit).

The Role of Public Welfare Services

In this rapidly changing situation, the public welfare services have a vital role to play, even if this will not necessarily be the same in every Member State. Diversity in the form, content and delivery of public services is the overriding characteristic of the European Union scene. Taking 'public welfare services' as defined in the introduction to mean those provided by governments (central and local) for social protection of their populations, patterns of delivery have developed in different ways over time in different countries (we illustrate these differences in greater detail in Chapter 2). In the post war period, most of the European welfare states passed through a period of rapid expansion, followed by a reassessment after the shock of the rise in the cost of energy in 1973 and the pressures of economic recession over the rest of that decade. Different countries responded differently: some consolidated their welfare systems; others embarked on substantial programmes of reform, some of which were aimed at reducing expenditure on welfare.

However, there are two key features which are common to every system. First, all of them are in a state of flux, in part as a result of the changes that have already been described. Second, all involve a variety of different actors: there are no welfare systems in the Union in which the State is wholly dominant or wholly absent. The responsibility for social welfare ultimately rests with governments but implementation is divided in distinctive national patterns between central and local governments, the market, formal and informal voluntary associations and individual citizens. So, in considering the present and future role of the public welfare services, it is important not to lose sight of the importance of the changing form of the relationships between public sector bodies and other service delivery agencies.

12

Pressures for Change

There are a number of reasons why the role of public welfare services has been changing at an increasingly rapid pace:

.   pressures to reduce the **costs** of public services;
.   pressures to meet **increased needs** generated by social and economic changes;
.   pressures to improve the **efficiency and effectiveness** of services;
.   pressures to provide an **enhanced role for the users** of services and their representatives.

To a greater or lesser extent in Member States, one result of these pressures has been to open up a debate about the public services and to stimulate a process of change to adapt public services to these new circumstances, especially in the context of reductions in public resources.

Some people would argue that these developments, taken together, amount to a crisis in delivery of public welfare. In order to understand the nature of the situation with which the providers and consumers of public services are now confronted, it is necessary to look more closely at all these sources of pressure.

The increase in the **costs of services** has generated a widespread perception that the 'burden of welfare' has become too great for the economies of individual countries to bear. The increase has been driven by a number of linked factors: the high cost, social as well as economic, of increased unemployment and the poverty associated with it and costs stemming from other social and demographic changes. The numbers of those reliant on public welfare services have consequently increased; and there have also been increases in the demands generated by rising expectations among consumers and articulated by the users of services and pressure groups acting for them.

Demographic change and in particular the ageing of the European population poses difficult challenges. Different countries have reacted to these challenges in a variety of ways; some by measures designed to economise on the cost of providing services - for example by cutting or capping expenditure on welfare or changing the rules for eligibility for receipt of services or benefits (eg, raising the age at which citizens qualify for pensions).

These developments have also placed a high premium on measures designed to improve the **efficiency and effectiveness of public welfare services** - what is sometimes described as 'the new public management'. This has stemmed partly from scepticism about the capacity of these services to cope, particularly under increased pressure, and partly from a desire to make them more responsive to the public. This has necessarily involved rethinking the role of departments and agencies, the ways in which they present themselves to consumers of their services and also organisational patterns and the distribution of responsibilities for service delivery. At one end of the spectrum comes privatisation of functions by devolving responsibility for delivery of services wholly or partly to the market.

The objective of these reforms has been not just to deliver services in a more efficient way but also to make them **more responsive to consumers** - both by providing better information about the services being delivered and also to improve quality. Attempts have also been made to encourage involvement of users in the planning and processes of service delivery. These aims also reflect the influence of consumer movements, increased emphasis on satisfaction of individual wants, growing diversity of the population and the wide range of demands generated within it, both individual and collective (EFILWC, 1990). Additional pressure for change has also come from below, from the consumers themselves and through locally-based community action, as illustrated in the report 'Out of the Shadows', which forms part of the Foundation's rolling programme of research and policy analysis in the area of social cohesion (EFILWC, 1992).

These developments are taking place in a large number of countries, both inside and outside the European Union (OECD, 1994). However, it is important to stress that they are not all taking place simultaneously across all countries of the Union or at a uniform tempo; there are wide variations in policy and outcome both between and within different countries.

In this process of change it is important to reconcile economic and social objectives and to see public services as both a means of sustaining social cohesion and also as a player with a vital role in economic development. As the Economic and Social Committee's Opinion has it, "an efficient and effective public service and a good supporting infrastructure are important for the further development of the internal market" (1993). The public sector also plays a key role as an employer; ECOSOC estimates that, on a broad definition of the public sector, it employs almost 25m people (15% of the economically active population) across the Union. This underlines the importance of the involvement of the social partners - the employers and trades unions - in debates about the future strategic role of the public services, and in addressing the issues outlined above. It should also acknowledge the three-fold concern of employers from the private sector in public services: as "corporate citizens" with social responsibilities; as contributors to social security; and as providers of services in the context of privatisation. Trades unions too are concerned with the quality of services and their effectiveness, as well as employment levels, working conditions and morale of staff within the public sector (European Public Services Committee, 1994).

The debates currently taking place - to which this report contributes - raise a series of basic issues: for example, how services can be targeted with maximum effectiveness in use of resources to support those most in need without stigmatising or even segregating them. Some of the solutions now being adopted modify the role of public services in ways which fundamentally affect the relationship between State and Citizen. In the course of the Foundation's research a number of key themes have been defined that both relate to these broader issues and also engage in a practical way with situations on the ground.

Key Themes for Policy Development

. the need for the public services to make **special provision for those in most need** - the socially excluded who - because of their particular circumstances, are likely to be especially dependent on public services to sustain themselves and their families and to assist in their economic and social reintegration. They are also usually the people with least capacity for exercising control over their relationship with the providers of services and therefore most in need of new means of asserting their rights; they are at risk of being politically as well as socially excluded, either because they fail to exercise their political rights or because as non-citizens they do not possess them;

. the need to view and assess public service change strategies from **the perspective of all the interested parties** - policy-makers, management, workers involved in delivering the services, users of services, citizens and taxpayers - so that all obtain benefits in change;

. the need to take account of the **situation of women** who are the main front-line providers and the main users of public welfare services, yet are under-represented in the policy making and management arenas: the equal opportunities dimension of public sector change.

In reviewing the experience of change on the ground in consumer-oriented and quality based initiatives, the Foundation's research explored the level of awareness of these key issues, as well as examining the impact of these changes in public services. As will shortly be clear, there is often a surprising lack of recognition of the importance of these issues both in the change process itself and in the wider policy debate.

Summary and Conclusions

In this Chapter we have set out the essential background to recent changes in the public welfare sector in the EU. Changes in the economic, social and demographic context are briefly reviewed and their impact on future social cohesion established. The resulting pressures for change in the public welfare services have been to reduce costs, meet increased needs, improve efficiency and effectiveness and provide an enhanced role for consumers. Three key themes for development in public welfare services are underlined: the importance of making specific provision for the socially excluded; the need to involve all the significant actors in the processes of change and the special relevance of the role of women.

CHAPTER TWO :   The Dynamics of Change

The developments taking place across Europe and described in the first Chapter of this report imply an urgent need for further action, in which the public welfare services must necessarily play a prominent part. However, the diversity of traditions and practices in the various welfare systems, to which reference has already been made (Chapter 1) means that responses to the challenges faced by all European countries have taken a wide variety of different forms. In order to understand and learn from these responses it is helpful to establish the key characteristics of the different systems in the eight countries of the EU in which the Foundation's research has been conducted (Denmark, France, Germany, Greece, Ireland, Italy, Portugal and the UK).

A wide variety of different reform programmes and initiatives are already underway in these countries, many of which will be described in greater detail later in the report. The brief summary descriptions that follow set these initiatives in their national context. It is important to emphasise that not only do these different national systems possess different characteristics but the trajectory of change within them has also been very different.

Eight National Welfare Systems : Some Key Characteristics

In **Germany,** the welfare services reflect a pattern based on legislation which confers on workers an enforceable legal right to welfare; but participation in decision making is structured on an institutional basis - there is little external pressure to make the public services more consumer-sensitive. The basic operating principle is subsidiarity; each level of government intervenes in welfare delivery only where other agencies (including the family) have failed. Charitable associations are paid to deliver the majority of social services. 'Empowerment' has been widely debated but is conceived of in terms of access rather than passing of control or influence over services to consumers.

In **France,** the model is a centralised public welfare service with the State taking the major share of responsibility for delivery. This in turn means that the State is a major employer and trades unions are important players: women make up the majority of public sector workers. Debate about modernisation of bureaucratic

---

public services and decentralisation of delivery has taken hold latterly and produced a sequence of reforms, including the introduction of a public services charter. The main focus of the move towards change has been to secure improvements in information, co-ordination of services and *acceuil*. Very little progress has been made yet with securing direct consumer involvement and there is no national consumer movement directly relating to public services, although there are a number of associations promoting the interests of excluded groups.

The **United Kingdom** has experienced very rapid change in the 1980s. Here, the move has been towards reducing the scope of State provision and introducing the concept of 'enabling'. This term implies contracting out of an increasing proportion of public welfare services to independent and private sector agencies. Concern for consumers has been an increasing preoccupation of local authorities, whose direct service delivery functions have declined. The executive agencies 'hived off' from central government departments to take responsibility for delivery of cash services and benefits have also taken up issues of sensitivity to customers. Charters have been devised to codify the entitlements of users of individual services; these have been brought together in the form of the Citizen's Charter (which does not however confer rights).

Ireland is a hybrid case, showing some influence of UK experience. This is a rapidly evolving welfare system, which was originally heavily dependent on the voluntary sector and specifically the Catholic church but is now increasingly dominated by statutory provision centrally organised. Local government has only a very limited role. There has been a similar sequence of public service reforms, which have focused specifically on social rights and attempt to provide a consumer orientation for the public sector as a whole. Charters are also a feature of the Irish system; and some key agencies have a clear set of consumer-led objectives. The National Economic and Social Forum has recently presented a major report recommending quality improvements in social services (NESF, 1995).

Italy is another mixed case. The welfare system is best described as fragmented, with economic goals predominating over social ones but with a lack of cost control and an endemic lack of co-ordination within the system, which is also characterised by patronage and waste. Popular demand has been a powerful driving force for change; and the fragmentation of the system has left 'spaces' to be colonised by local and regional level initiatives. 'New Management' programmes, often based on the use of new technology, are quite frequently encountered; there have also been a number of examples of local citizens' charters.

Denmark is the only example of a 'social democratic' model in the group, although the public welfare system is a comparatively new development, associated with the country's late industrialisation. Unlike experience in most of the other countries studied, local government has played a central role in recent developments in the public welfare system, with independent access to resources through local taxation. Decentralisation has been a major theme of reform over the 1980s, coupled with strong pressure on the public sector to be more productive. The 'free municipality' movement has some limited experience with privatisation. Consumer involvement has been seen as an important objective but difficult to achieve in practice, posing problems both for consumers and staff.

Portugal has experienced modernisation which arrived late but with a rush, as part of the process of democratisation. Vigorous attempts have been made to 'de bureaucratise' a very traditional system which displayed only minimal sensitivity to the needs of the consumers of services. This new approach seeks to establish through public services reforms a new relationship between state and citizens and has been led from the top. Public service charters and the use of new technology have played a considerable part in this process. Local experiment has also been facilitated; but the influence of consumers is very limited; the system is still largely based on the traditional resources of family and Church, together with a decentralised public welfare service.

Greece shared with Portugal during the post-war period the experience of dictatorship and a highly traditional public service bureaucracy dominated by paper-pushing. Welfare has traditionally depended upon the family; local authorities have had only a marginal role and professional social services have not been fully developed. The State has provided benefits, but at a low level. Public sector reform has been imposed top-down and has not been service specific. Despite the reform programmes, some of them making use of new technology, new initiatives have had to make their way through a highly centralised system in which bureau managers have low status and little power; innovation often depends upon organisations operating outside the state. Consumers have also tended to be passive and limited in their expectations, complaining about the low level of benefits, rather than quality of service.

Commentary: The Key Actors in Change

As this summary suggests, each of the countries studied has passed through changes, in the course of which different actors and institutions have played different roles. In some systems, the main driving force for change comes predominantly from the centre: Ireland and Italy, for different reasons, fit that pattern. In other systems, local government performs a much more developed function: Germany (with its unique Federal pattern of governance), Denmark, where local government enjoys a high level of autonomy and increasingly France where decentralisation has been introduced on a substantial scale. In all these cases, however, key functions are retained at the centre. In other cases, like

Portugal and Greece, the role of local government in welfare services having barely developed, the responsibility for innovation has necessarily rested with central government or its local agencies. In the United Kingdom, by contrast, the role of local authorities, once dominant in delivery of public welfare services, is under review and their role as direct providers is now substantially reduced.

In addition, a substantial role is played in some countries by organisations operating partly or wholly outside the State: the churches, voluntary welfare associations and small-scale community and self help groups. Examples are the case of Germany, where the highly developed system of subsidiarity in service delivery is especially striking; also the growth of the *économie sociale* in France and the increased role played by the voluntary sector in the welfare services in the UK. Even in Denmark, with its well-developed tradition of State responsibility for delivery, a degree of pluralism is now beginning to appear. In the 'emergent' systems, such as Greece, the State has never fully developed its role as a provider of welfare services, even though the voluntary sector is weak. Ireland and Portugal are hybrid cases, with the central State playing a major role but the churches still taking on a significant (although diminishing) share of the responsibilities. Finally, the role of small-scale, informal bodies remains a major if under publicised source of welfare in all eight countries and the family (predominantly women within families) continues to be the largest resource of all.

At the same time, the market is becoming more important as a source of social welfare; in some countries, this is partly a reversion to past patterns, in others it is a new development driven by the search for efficiency and cost effectiveness (the UK is the pioneer here but there is some evidence of similar developments elsewhere, for example in the Netherlands). Where the State does retain overall responsibility - such as in the provision of pensions - market-type devices have often been introduced into the procedures for delivering services.

In all the countries studied it has usually been the central government that has been the chief actor in introducing (though not necessarily in implementing) change. This concentration of responsibility at the centre means that it is of particular importance that policies and programmes to improve the responsiveness of public welfare services to citizens and consumers should be an explicit priority for national governments.

In fact, ambitious programmes of reform feature in almost all the countries studied. A range of devices have been employed to address the problems of over-bureaucratization and insensitivity to consumer demands: new agencies, new policies and procedures, Charters and observatories (UK, Portugal, France). These programmes vary as between different countries, both in their content and the manner in which they have been introduced. These contrasts have a great deal to do with the baseline from which action has been launched. For example, in the 'emergent' welfare systems governments have found themselves undertaking complex reforms without previous experience and with limited capacity. The need for modernisation has been clearly grasped, especially in the case of Portugal; but the means to achieve it have often been lacking. Ambitious public sector reform programmes have been launched in France and Germany - the latter complicated by the impact of reunification after 1991; the issues here have been around the need to modify well-established institutions and procedures and the action has been taken at both central and local level.

The UK is perhaps the most radical example of change introduced from the centre. For some while, there has been general agreement that the public services were over bureaucratic in their functioning and tended to be dominated by professional interests. However, the Government's reforms have proved controversial. The basic dispute has been over the ultimate structure desired: whether to move towards a residual model of provision, in which the responsibility for delivering services is shifted into the private or independent sectors emphasising market-related objectives (which is the view being promoted by central government), or retain a substantial role for the public sector (as many local authorities would prefer).

These changes have confronted the State as employer with a series of difficult challenges. Given that the State sector of welfare is a major source of employment in most of the countries studied, the content of the changes being made and the ways in which they have been introduced carry with them a considerable potential for conflict. Many of the new programmes designed to slim down bureaucracy and reduce public expenditure have also implied a threat of job losses. The reaction of public sector unions to such changes and their willingness to consider trading off these losses against the enhanced job satisfaction that the changes can also produce is a potentially important element in many of these situations. The reform process presupposes not only consensus about objectives but a willingness on all sides to engage in constructive dialogue in the interests of longer term benefits for all the different parties involved - consumers, staff and employers.

Key Content of Changes

The responsibility for innovation is quite widely distributed across the eight countries studied; so is the content of the programmes that have been introduced. For present purposes these initiatives can be divided into seven broad categories:

*   General innovations based on 'the new public management';

*   The introduction of new technology;

*   Privatisation and 'learning from business';

*   Decentralisation and devolving responsibilities to localities;

*   Pluralism in service delivery;

*   Expansion of consumer rights;

*   Equal opportunities policies.

The distribution of these policies at national level in public welfare services across the eight case study countries has been plotted in the following table:

TABLE 2.1	Distribution of national policy initiatives							
	DK	FR	DE	GR	IRL	I	P	UK
New management	X	X	X	X	X	(X)	X	X
New technology	X	X	X	(X)	X	(X)	(X)	X
Private sector techniques		(X)						X
Decentralisation	X	X	X	(X)		(X)		
Pluralism in delivery	(X)	X	X		(X)			X
Enhanced consumer rights		(X)	(X)	(X)	(X)		(X)	(X)
Equal opportunities								(X)

X   = fully present
(X)   = present in part

Discussion: Significance of National Policy Initiatives

Each of the terms used requires some elaboration; the following section defines them in more detail and establishes their relevance.

New Public Management is an all-embracing term for a group of public sector reforms, encompassing initiatives designed to restructure and reorient the public services in order to achieve greater efficiency and effectiveness in service delivery, better value for money and a better quality outcome which offers more choice to the consumer of services (OECD 1994, op cit). In the British context, for example, it has been defined as: 'a focus on management, not policies and on performance appraisal and efficiency; the disaggregation of public bureaucracies into agencies which deal with each other on a user-pay basis.... and a style of management which emphasises, among other things, output targets, limited term contracts and freedom to manage' (Rhodes 1991).

Such a comprehensive programme of reform, where it has been attempted, poses challenges to the management of public service organisations and to the staff. Both have to rethink their role and their relationship with the consumers of the services they are providing. It requires clear thinking about the objectives of organisations and the means by which those objectives are best met and the ways in which performance is measured. It also raises questions about the skills and level of staffing required and the motivation and morale of staff - issues on which the public sector unions have an important contribution to make.

There is little doubt that the introduction of **new technology** can be a powerful instrument in giving consumers better access to services and improving the quality of the service itself (the experience of the modernisation of many private services - banking and insurance - reinforces the point). It is also one of the preconditions for the introduction of some of the key elements of the new public administration - for example, introduction of budgets broken down to the level of subordinate 'cost centres' and the ready availability of data for constructing performance indicators. The cost of providing the equipment (typically, PCs and modern telecommunications facilities) is no longer very great; the main investment will be in staff training. The gain here is not only in the more efficient service it will help to provide but also in the enhanced sense of worth enjoyed by the staff concerned. But this type of reform eventually depends for its full effect on a fundamental change in the working environment and perhaps the culture in which it is set. If the practice of the agency is not open to scrutiny by outsiders (both the users of the service and those who fund it) and properly accountable - 'transparent' is the term usually employed - then sophisticated technology will not of itself do the job.

Private sector techniques or 'learning from business' is also controversial, at least in part because of concern that the 'public sector ethos' and social goals will be undermined by an attempt to simulate market conditions. Some of the management techniques adapted from private sector use hold out promise of substantial efficiency gains; but they are essentially about process, not outcomes. Clarification of the objectives that are being served is essential; in this context, Professor Bent Greve comments that:

".....the immediate answer we get in the public debate is, we have to learn from the market economy, and therefore tools are created for measuring efficiency and making cost benefit analysis and so on, which in many respects is all right, but it is not the answer to the problems of inefficiency in the public sector because it is not because they are doing things inefficiently that we have problems." (Danish National Institute for Social Research, 1992:21).

In other words, pressures generated by private sector techniques - the push towards greater efficiency and parsimony in the use of resources - need to be balanced by the need to be demonstrably fair and honest in the use to which public funds are put.

These comments raise the question of whether there are values intrinsic to the public welfare services and particular relationships between public agencies and their consumers which could be compromised by the introduction of commercial procedures and market values. Core values such as equity and basic entitlements to a range of quality services not rationed by cost could be put at risk. There are, at the least, dangers attached to an unthinking rush towards modernisation which does not take account of the nature of the service involved and the relationship between the State and people both as individuals and in their social networks.

Decentralisation is properly seen as a major element in the reform of public services - an application in practice of the principle of subsidiarity, devolving responsibilities to the level at which they can be most effectively discharged. In the neighbourhood, public services can link with informal provision within local communities to meet needs in the form and in the terms in which the recipients of services choose (EFILWC, 1992). But two qualifications need to be noted; first, a significant degree of control over resources needs to be devolved with the responsibility for delivery of services - otherwise it is just a matter of implementing decisions taken higher up the line and devolving responsibility for 'saying no nicely'. Administrative measures for local delivery on terms laid down from the centre in that style are not really decentralisation (the preferred term for these measures is 'de-concentration'). Secondly, there should be some element of democratic decision-taking; otherwise, there is a risk that unaccountable organisations may neglect the legitimate interests of disadvantaged or under-represented minorities. Democratic accountability may also provide some protection for staff concerned about the risks of delegated responsibility or becoming 'too close to the client' (EFILWC, 1990).

Welfare pluralism - the delivery of services by a wider variety of agencies, with government acting as the funder of services and thereafter confining itself to performing the additional roles of regulation and inspection - is well established in many EU countries. In others, the process of developing from state-delivered welfare services to more diverse systems, often through the use of contracts, is now well advanced. One virtue of this approach is that the consumer who is in the right place, with sufficient resources, may have a wider range of choices. Another is the presumption that increased competition will help to improve quality and keep down costs. However, difficulties may arise in practice (asymmetries of knowledge and power between purchasers and providers) which put potential gains for consumers at risk and diminish their opportunities to take part in decision making. Service provision by local community groups may approximate more closely to expressed needs but raise issues about quality of service and accountability (EFILWC 1992). This approach is also problematic when reforms are introduced with the intention (explicit or covert) of securing economies in public expenditure, while high transition and transaction costs may limit the effects of competition and innovation.

These difficulties give added significance to the growing array of mechanisms by which performance can be measured and people held to account for performance. They include the battery of means by which politically accountable public bodies can monitor and enforce performance of their agents - performance targets, regulation and inspection of standards, contract specification and enforcement. They also include the mechanisms by which individual consumers can hold providers to account, including legal entitlements, charters, complaints systems and ombudsmen.

Accountability to individual service users is closely linked to political accountability, since the pursuit of private grievance is often the means by which public issues are made public. However, these mechanisms are frequently fragile, especially when they depend on the protests of vulnerable individuals who depend, over a long period, on the providers about whom they are complaining. They also vary with the particular type of welfare system which is dominant - some giving entitlements to users and others giving limited discretion to providers.

The **expansion of consumer rights** is another active area of reform. The initiatives taken in most EU countries during the course of the 1980s to make welfare services more user-friendly and secure better redress for grievances have now, inter alia, generated: a set of Charters setting out the entitlements of users (Belgium, France, Portugal and the UK); Ombudsman services, such as in France and Ireland; and a public sector 'quality observatory' in Spain. The OECD in their review of recent developments in public service management have also identified four distinct objectives that reforms would need to satisfy in order to produce a genuinely client-centred service: greater transparency; statements of entitlements; identifying and satisfying specific client requirements; and improved accessibility (OECD, 1994). Charters provide a useful focus for this type of action; but, as we shall see, it is an open question whether they actually provide the consumers of services with significant additional rights, as opposed to a convenient means of securing remedies.

Equal opportunity policies, finally, are a necessary but not a sufficient condition for securing provision of equal quality for users from diverse and disadvantaged sectors of the population. In addition to the extension of rights and opportunities to women as service users and providers, policies in this area need to address the inequalities and obstacles faced by all consumers of public services in consequence of their ethnicity, age, disability or sexuality. Moreover, to provide the same service to all users may not produce equity in outcomes.

In developing the equal opportunities dimension of their services, public welfare agencies need to recognise that approaches that create specialist services for disadvantaged consumers may result in increasing rather than decreasing the stigmatisation and marginalisation of individuals, groups in society and communities. Disability movements in the EU and their campaigns for civil rights have provided an important reminder of this danger. The promotion of greater equality in rights, entitlements to public welfare services and opportunities also needs to engage with the broader issues of citizenship.

The National Policy Balance Sheet

In summary, the effects of the introduction of the various different types of policies described and their consequences could be divided between **opportunities** and **constraints.** These are interconnected, so that each opportunity for taking new initiatives had its mirror-image in obstacles that may impede them or qualify their success.

TABLE 2.2	Opportunities	Constraints
New public management	Efficiency gains; value for money	Job losses in public agencies; fragmentation and accountability problems
Introduction of new technology	Requirement for higher skills; empowerment of staff	Cost of training
Private sector techniques	Application of business skills	Inappropriate values?
Decentralisation	Devolved responsibility; sensitivity to local circumstances	Fragmentation; need to define core values
Pluralism in delivery	Variety and choice for consumers	Loss of wider accountability
Consumer rights	Empowering consumers	Insufficient basis for remedies
Equal opportunities	Access for excluded	Stigmatisation; separate provision

The current European Union policy environment

Action that has been taken at European level provides an additional element in the overall policy framework. The agenda still tends to be dominated, as the EU moves out of recession, by the concerns about cost of providing welfare and the pressures generated by demographic change. The Commission has commented that:

"Governments may be tempted to avoid being caught in... distributional conflict between the generations and may therefore wish to promote private social security provision. However, private provision will only develop to the extent that public provision is reduced, which will, of course, be hugely unpopular" (European Commission, 1993:22).

Co-ordinated action to address this, and other major issues presents a number of practical difficulties. The evolution of a concerted European social policy is proving to be a long drawn out process (Kleinman and Piachaud, 1993). Opportunities are constrained by limitations on the competence of the Commission to act in this area; and much of the social action in the pre-Maastricht period has related specifically to the labour market (in particular, training) and has only indirectly addressed some of the key questions which are likely to determine future patterns of social protection in the EU.

However, labour market policies are crucial, to the extent that unemployment and its impact is central to current changes and one of the main determining factors in creating and perpetuating social exclusion. But policies in this area are also controversial in that they define a sharp division between those who have promoted the notion that the key to finding solutions is through deregulation of the market, increasing 'wage flexibility', reforms in unemployment benefit and constraining the role of trades unions (cf the UK Government's statement, Competitiveness and Employment (1994)) and those who view the flexible labour market as the prelude to 'social dumping' and are keen to preserve the European social model. These policies are therefore controversial; the Commission's White Paper on Growth, Competitiveness and Employment draws particular attention to the need for policy to reflect wider concerns -"the need to maintain social and industrial peace, and to avoid creating further poverty among those groups already in the weakest position on the labour market" and to the danger that attempts to reduce the level of job protection will lead ".....to the growth of two-tier labour markets - those with secure permanent jobs and those with insecure temporary jobs. Pressure to increase labour market flexibility without countervailing actions has, moreover, often reduced

31

rather than increased the incentives for firms and individuals to invest in much needed training and retraining" (European Commission, 1993b:29).

There are unresolved disagreements in this field, notably the UK's non-adherence to the Social Charter (December 1989, properly the 'Community Charter of Fundamental Social Rights for Workers') and the opt-out negotiated by the UK government in 1991 from the Social Chapter of the Maastricht Treaty (which provides for EU actions to support and complement of Member States' activities in protecting workers' health and safety, working conditions, informing and consulting workers, equal opportunity and treatment and integration of people excluded from the labour market). Their response to the consultative process on the European Commission's Green Paper on Social Policy (EC1994b) suggests that the UK's position on European social policies will remain unchanged for the immediate future.

Nevertheless, a suite of special programmes addressing social issues (in the broadest sense) is now in place, developed over quite a long period. Examples are the successive actions taken under the Structural Funds (specifically the Social and Regional Funds and Community initiatives such as HORIZON, NOW, EMPLOYMENT); demonstration projects on a far smaller scale undertaken as part of the Commission's own action and research programmes - for example the three successive European programmes to combat poverty, the HELIOS programme for people with disabilities, the IRIS programme for vocational training for women - designed as catalysts to disseminate information and good practice at local and national level; and the creation of the observatories to monitor policy developments in certain specific sectors (poverty, the family, elderly, employment).

In July 1994, the Commission published their Social Policy White Paper. This contains detailed proposals for further interventions in the labour market, including targets for basic skills, a job guarantee for all under 18s, a revival of apprenticeships and better information and consultation of employees. This is an enterprise in which the social partners - the representatives of both sides of industry, whose role is becoming increasingly significant in this area - are to be involved. Additional measures to promote equality of opportunity are also foreshadowed, including steps to improve skills and professional qualifications and to make child care facilities more widely available. Finally, further initiatives to develop a European model of welfare, to address the problems of poverty and to re-integrate excluded groups and combat discrimination on grounds of age and disability are also foreseen; it is proposed, from 1996, to publish an annual 'Equality Report' monitoring progress under these heads (European Commission, 1994).

Taken together with the other initiatives summarised above, the Social Policy White Paper represents a significant step towards the devising of a coherent European social policy, which would provide a basis for addressing some of the main issues with which this report is concerned. This has been reinforced by the recent publication of the Medium-Term Social Action Programme 1995-1997 (European Commission, 1995).

Summary and Conclusions

In this chapter we have provided a summary account of some of the main characteristics of the public welfare services in the eight EU countries selected for study and recent changes that have taken place within them. Seven key facets of those changes were identified: the introduction of new public management and new technology; privatisation; decentralisation; pluralism in service delivery, the recognition of consumer rights and equal opportunity policies. These policies and the opportunities and constraints attached to each of them have been explored in further detail. This account of the national policy context has also been set in the context of the development of European social policies, leading up to the Social Policy White Paper of 1994 and the Medium-Term Social Action Programme 1995-1997.

CHAPTER THREE :   Models for Change in Public Welfare Services

The importance of involving consumers more closely in the planning and delivery of public welfare services has now become more generally recognised. It is an element of the reorientation in national policy discussed in the last chapter. However, the precise objectives to be served by doing so and the outcomes that should be achieved often remain vague. Even the terms in common use in the debate are often confusing and imprecise. For example, politicians of both left and right have fastened on to the concept of 'empowerment'; but it is clear from the contexts in which they have employed it that they mean very different things when they use the term. As Gaster and Taylor have commented:

"The words 'partnership', 'empowerment', 'consumer' and 'citizen' have been worked very hard in recent years and can easily give rise to scepticism. They raise questions of rights and power, exclusion and equality, of representativeness and representation, which could easily be side-tracked in organisations more concerned with form than content, with rhetoric than reality. For some, they suggest a move to better marketing and the adoption of the consumerism adopted by the commercial world; for others they suggest a move from representative to a more participative democracy." (Local Government Management Board, 1993).

This chapter sets out to clarify the main objectives for consumer involvement and the terms on which it can be achieved.

Stages of Consumer Involvement

Some people have found it helpful to conceive of the process of involvement as a continuous one, which takes place in a sequence of defined stages. For example, the OECD in their recent report on public services suggest that there may be a continuum of client involvement and client discretion with five identifiable stages. This is sometimes referred to as a 'ladder of participation' (Arnstein, 1971):

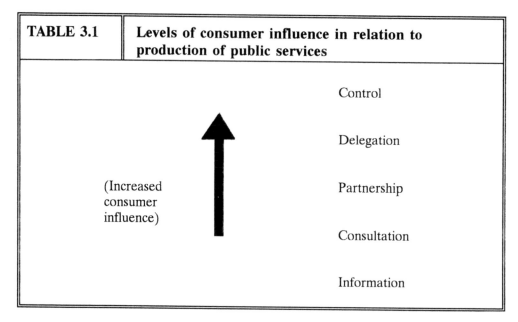

TABLE 3.1	Levels of consumer influence in relation to production of public services

(Increased consumer influence)

Control

Delegation

Partnership

Consultation

Information

(OECD, 1994)

The problem is that while this diagram tells a useful story it does not give us the whole picture. There are various problems: first, that it focuses on administrative structures and processes and therefore assesses the users' benefits from the changing situation in institutional terms. Second, the sequence of transactions does not take full account of the different roles in which a consumer may relate to the public welfare services. Third, it suggests a transition by stages, moving logically upwards from one level to the next. This takes little account of the nature of the different services, some providing cash benefits on strict rules of entitlement (eg, pensions), and others delivering care in ways that may involve joint production by 'providers' and 'consumers'. Finally, the form in which the sequence is usually presented also implies that the process operates only in the direction of increased 'empowerment'. Experience suggests that this is not always the case. It is also important to recognise that the scope and importance of the different levels varies with the type of service.

Better information made freely available may be a sufficient end in itself - providing all that consumers require to satisfy their needs - and what happens at the final stage of the process may have little to do with empowerment of consumers. Delegating responsibility for control over delivery of a service may simply be a device for cutting costs and shedding responsibility for the quality of the service being delivered (EFILWC, 1992). Consumers from excluded groups may find themselves disadvantaged at all stages of the process by lack of power and the absence of relevant skills. And, as Christofferson and Hanson (1994) point out in their report on Denmark, the crucial issue of resource allocation cuts across the whole concept of a steady rise through stages. Reforms may be checked or put into reverse by shortage of crucial resources (financial and human) at the moment of 'ripe time'. If, on arrival at the top of the ladder, these resources are not available, the climb will have been in vain.

The individual (or group) in their role as consumer will have difficulty in confronting many of these issues; but in their role as citizen they can and should be able to exert direct influence over events, in a democratic system. This role can be exercised either individually or collectively. However, not all citizens have equal access to the means of influencing decision making; and some consumers do not possess full citizen rights.

This raises the important issue of rights and the premise on which many of the public sector reforms are being undertaken - for example, the introduction of Charters in various European Union countries and the extent to which they confer rights on service users. As the OECD report points out, different countries' initiatives will reflect a wide range of issues:

"These fundamental issues include: how far do the rights of clients go, compared say to those of the taxpayer? Are we really talking about clients, in the sense of a market, or about citizens who also have obligations? Some see the reforms as resolving an inherent conflict between public servants and citizens in favour of the latter with a shift of power from the supplier to the client. Others see it in terms of the state's legitimacy being based on socially useful state activity. Some see the reforms as improving equality and democracy by recognising all clients (citizens) as having equal entitlements, thus obviating favouritism or corruption in the delivery of public services" (OECD 1994, op cit para 22).

The potential confusion of roles is well exemplified in the debates in the UK on the status of the Conservative Government's 'Citizen's Charter' which addresses many of these issues - by facilitating complaints and providing redress - but does so on the basis not of entitlements but as part of a dialogue between service providers and consumers designed to improve the efficiency and effectiveness of public agencies and enhance service quality. This is why critics prefer to refer to this document as a 'consumer's charter', in the sense that we have defined consumers in our glossary.

All this suggests that there is a need to conceive of the processes in two, linked forms and to distinguish clearly, as Gaster and Taylor argue "on the one hand between the individual and collective ways in which consumers and citizens may be involved, and, on the other, between the different levels of power and responsibility which may be given to them" (Local Government Management Board op cit:12).

Means of Involving Consumers

Equipped with this broader concept of the interlocking processes involved in the development of a consumer-oriented approach in the public services, we now turn to examine some of the key means which are being used to achieve greater responsiveness. These are distilled from earlier publications in the Foundation's research programme (EFILWC, 1990, 1992, 1994) and from discussions of the research group in the project. In broad terms, they could be summarised as follows:

Access: making services more readily available to consumers by bringing them closer through decentralisation of delivery to small-scale, locally based units both within and outside the public sector, by changing the style in which services are provided at the point of delivery (*acceuil*) and by ensuring that the service that is provided is fully integrated;

Choice: improving the consumers' situation by allowing them to exercise options, both within the service they are receiving and between alternative providers; and facilitating competition, where appropriate, to produce a wider range of options;

Voice: giving consumers the opportunity to express their views on the service they are receiving and where they are dissatisfied providing a response which meets their legitimate grievances; this links to

Accountability: providing the means by which those who deliver services are made responsible for the stewardship, both through improvements in information - greater 'transparency' in the operation of services - and by making existing democratic machinery more accessible.

Components of the Model

Access is properly the concern of consumers, in that the issue of the prompt and easy availability of services lies at the heart of the consumer movement's campaigns for reform. Services provided in the locality at the 'human scale' are almost by definition more accessible and this is particularly important for those tied to their immediate vicinity by limited mobility, lack of income and other domestic commitments. Hence the importance, already several times underlined, of decentralisation as a leading theme of reform. However, access relates to time and also to openness and acceptability, as well as space. The former is complicated by work patterns on both sides of the counter: local offices closed at "unsocial" hours may provide less access. The latter has particular resonance for excluded (even stigmatised) minorities who have a right to equally accepting and acceptable services which respect their identities. In these situations, management may require compromises and some untidiness in service patterns. It may also require the explicit, top-down statement of principles of access, and their monitoring. This becomes more important as localisation is frequently combined with delegated discretion to staff, so that the normal command and control structure may not be available to manage these tensions.

Choice is not simply a matter of providing alternative options at the point of delivery in order that consumers can have the opportunity to maximise their satisfaction through selecting the option that most closely corresponds with their preference. It also has to do with the basis on which any alternatives are offered; here, the citizen has a legitimate interest in the cost of providing a range of services and the social consequences of doing or not doing so.

In exercising that interest, citizens may be concerned to protect potential and future users (as opposed to current ones) and also those people likely to lose out if the means of creating choice also creates competition between users for the favoured service. Equally, they will need to weigh the possible fragmentation, lack of transparency, costs of co-ordination and risks of market failure inherent in some means of affording choice against the danger of inward looking monopolies in which provider interests dominate.

A second complication over the exercise of choice concerns those services which are consumed over long periods of time and which are frequently jointly produced by collaboration between 'user' and 'provider', characteristically, social care. Here, partnership models where provision is negotiated may have more to offer than choice at a single point of entry, although the possibility of opting out may be an important safeguard.

Voice is another area in which the interests of consumers may not always correspond with those of citizens. Consumers may often wish to express dissent about the way in which public services are delivered (complaints procedures) or to become involved in expressing views about ways in which they can be improved (forums, advocacy). They may do this either individually or collectively, though existing democratic mechanisms or in alternative forms of protest (demonstrations, civil disobedience). But they will necessarily have a particular, not a general interest in the services which they are obtaining; the citizen may legitimately take issue with the priority being accorded to that service, as opposed to other equally deserving or socially significant ones. Consumers and pressure groups or advocates acting on their behalf are only one voice in the political arena, where these claims have to be reconciled and those who shout loudest (or whisper in the right ears) may not always have the best case. Nonetheless, legitimate conflicts of interest are more readily acknowledged and disappointing outcomes accepted if people feel that their views have been properly taken into account. And within politically determined parameters of resources and entitlements, voice can provide a powerful means of healthy dissent and debate.

Such issues connect with **accountability,** where the distinction between the responsibility for 'policy-making' and for 'implementation' is rarely clear-cut. Of course, in a democratic system it is ministers, mayors and other elected officials who are accountable to citizens through the electoral chain of command. This blunt but important safeguard needs to be retained where functions are split off into satellite agencies. Stating explicit terms and targets in the arrangements made when those agencies are established is an important means of retaining political accountability. However, policy-making through implementation causes some attenuation of this accountability. For example, managers, not ministers have become the victims when they failed to meet politically established performance targets within impossibly tight resource constraints.

The line of accountability becomes harder to follow where public funding is used to provide welfare through independent or commercial bodies, which is increasingly taking place in several European Union countries (see Chapter 2). This is not only because they may be less open to public scrutiny, but also because, in extreme versions it may be impossible to determine responsibility for actions in a complex chain of contractual relations - transparency in transactions has disappeared. There are also risks of confusion or even conflict when voluntary sector providers also attempt to perform a campaigning role.

Smith and Lipsky , in their 'Non-Profits For Hire' (1993) describe an American route to hell, paved with the good intentions of limiting government and promoting market efficiency in welfare services. Services are sub-contracted; public officials, mindful of the need to enforce proper accountability and probity, develop complex and detailed regulations, which add greatly to costs, make their job of monitoring and enforcement impossibly large; neither efficiency, not quality, nor robust financially healthy services are achieved; and the officials cannot afford the political consequences of openness.

These issues highlight the need for striking a balance between formal and informal means of establishing people's entitlements and making them real. They also point to the need to keep accountability systems closely interlinked with other mechanisms, such as performance indicators, voice and participation. Then the scope for debate, exploration, negotiation and re-interpretation - leading to a consensus among the partners which better fits their common purpose - is enhanced.

In the next chapter, we move on to relate the ideal models of change set out in this chapter to practical experience of ways in which changes are occurring on the ground, as revealed in the case studies undertaken in eight European Union countries.

Summary and Conclusions

This Chapter has identified various different types of consumer involvement, and examined the case for setting them out as a sequence, with defined stages of progressively greater involvement ('Arnstein's Ladder'). Our conclusion is that the process is better seen as one involving various different types of benefit for consumers; the four that seem most significant are access, voice, choice and accountability. Some of the general issues associated with these different aspects of involvement are identified and briefly reviewed as a preliminary to addressing the evidence from the case studies.

CHAPTER FOUR :   Experience on the Ground in Consumer-Oriented Action

This chapter draws upon the sixteen case studies of consumer-oriented initiatives which were undertaken: two in each of the eight countries chosen for the study. The basis for the selection of these case studies is explained in the introduction. They were intended to show how access for consumers of services can be improved, and how effective the different means of increasing their involvement, that have been developed, have proved to be in practice, given the different emphases in the various reform programmes studied. The case studies were also selected to illustrate the effects of change for managers and workers, as well as to enable examination of the implications related to equal opportunities and social exclusion.

Table 4.1 attempts to capture some of the range and richness of the resulting material. It describes the types of service and the type of agency involved, showing that, in this set of welfare initiatives, the payment of pensions and benefits were the most common subjects of change, but examples of health, social care and housing and employment services were also represented. The range of agencies involved was equally diverse.

TABLE 4.1	The case studies: which services and which agencies?		
Service Agencies	Housing & Employment	Social Services & Health	Benefits & Pensions
CENTRAL			ITALIAN Pensione Subito
State		.	GREEK IKA Pensions
			IRISH Quality Improvement Programme
Voluntary		ITALIAN Patients' Rights Tribunals	
SINGLE LOCAL			
Branch of National Agency		PORTUGUESE Beja Health project	UK Severnside Benefits Office
			IRISH Ballyfermot One- Stop Shop
			PORTUGUESE Amadora Social Security Office
Local authority	FRENCH Nantes Habitat	GREEK Kapi Older People's Centres	GERMAN Prosoz, Bremen
MULTI-AGENCY led by local authority		DANISH Odense Integrated Care for the Elderly	
		FRENCH l'Alliance	
		UK Wiltshire Community Care Users' Network	
Independent	GERMAN Rostock Arche		
	DANISH Hyldespjaeldet social network		

Content of Case Studies

In this section, we provide a brief account of the individual case studies, concentrating on the reasons why the schemes were introduced and the main lessons learned from them. Two of the studies are essentially concerned with reforms in the delivery of a major service at national level: these are the decentralisation of a large sector of the Greek pensions system and a parallel reform in the Italian system. A third provides comparable experience on the introduction of a modernised system of delivering cash benefits but at local authority level (Prosoz, Germany) and a fourth is specifically concerned with the delivery of benefits for a particular user group, persons claiming disability and sickness benefit (QUIP, Ireland).

Box A   Centrally directed reforms of single services

Pensione Subito (Italy)

The PS scheme was launched in 1990 by the Istituto Nazionale della Previdenza Sociale (INPS) the main official agency concerned with the delivery of pensions in Italy, as part of a series of reforms designed to improve the efficiency, productivity and quality of its services. The specific purpose of the PS scheme is to reduce the amount of time that people have to wait for payment of pensions, and by making offices accessible and involving people directly in the process of determining their own pension entitlements, to achieve 'added value' in the granting of benefits. It is also an exemplar of change, to be applied later to other sections.

The main innovative features of the scheme have been the use of new information technology, to decentralise decision-making and to enable one worker to deal with all aspects of payments to any one pensioner, thus improving the quality of the service and working conditions. The interactive dialogue with prospective pensioners gives them an active role the process of service delivery. Clear gains in efficiency are claimed, in terms of reduction of waiting times for pensions and easier access to localised offices.

Pension Award Decentralisation in Greek Social Security Agency (IKA)

This decentralisation scheme forms part of a range of similar initiatives introduced by the Greek Socialist Government during the 1980s. It is aimed at minimising the inconvenience caused to pension applicants using one of the main pension funds (IKA), through reducing excessive centralisation in the organisation of the service and speeding up the time taken to award pensions.

The scheme was experimental and took place in two rounds (1985-6 and from 1992 onwards) but only in a small number of offices; it was innovative, to the extent that it involved devolution of significant responsibilities to a level in the bureaucracy not previously entrusted with such tasks. Provisional assessments of the time taken to award pensions suggest that delivery time in decentralised offices has probably become marginally shorter and, more importantly, the level of user satisfaction has improved. However, the basis of the experiment is now being questioned, with suggestions that computerisation carried out at the centre is a more effective way of achieving the same objectives.

Box B   Local or specialised reform experiments

PROSOZ Benefits Scheme (Bremen, Germany)

Prosoz consists of the introduction of computer-supported, social security case-processing into local social security offices. The project was originally launched by the German Federal Ministry of Research in 1985 and taken up by the city of Bremen, which has responsibility for the delivery of these services and has been experiencing increased pressure through sharp rises in the numbers of cases. As in Italy, the special aspect of the project consists of the combined introduction of new technology in data processing with a reorganisation of the responsibilities of staff, who now provide a generic service to individuals. It was intended to overcome the fragmentation characteristic of the old system and deliver a cost-effective service which would also be more 'citizen-friendly'.

Evaluation suggests the change process took a long time, but that access to the services provided has been greatly improved and that there have been substantial gains in quality, so that it has become both faster and more flexible. Prosoz has also achieved considerable savings in costs. However, attempts by the users of services to become involved in the reform process have been only marginally successful, since the challenges presented by personnel issues have predominated.

Quality Improvement Programme (QUIP) Department of Social Welfare (Ireland)

QUIP was a pilot programme undertaken primarily to improve the quality and speed of service to clients claiming disability benefits from the General Benefits (and Sickness) Branch of the Department of Social Welfare. It was also intended to test the feasibility of a structured approach to quality improvement in a civil service context. QUIP was conceived of as an action-research project, carried out by six action teams composed of staff drawn from within the department. It was conducted in two phases between January 1989 and September 1990.

Among several gains claimed for the experiment are faster responses to new claims, faster payments of existing claims and simplification of procedures. Team members also reported gains in terms of their own experience and the opportunity to make a creative input into the process of redesigning the service. This suggests that quality improvement can be achieved by harnessing the experience and ideas of frontline and backline staff within quality teams.

These four studies are likely to be a source of lessons about the impact of the introduction of new technology, the resulting changes in the role of staff, and improvements in the quality of services, measured by speed and accuracy of delivery. However, they do not have much direct evidence to offer on the themes of user empowerment: they are about internal reforms to the official machinery, on a common agenda of bureaucratic modernisation, although this is important, particularly in countries with a lot of "red tape". At the other end of the range, in terms of style and size fall the small scale experimental action projects in Denmark and Rostock, in former East Germany. Both were conducted largely at local community level and used a variety of informal techniques designed to promote local involvement.

Box C   Local action projects

Hyldespjaeldet social network (Denmark)

Hyldespjaeldet is a non-profit rental housing estate in Albertslund Municipality, Greater Copenhagen. The action was initiated by the management group elected by the residents and had as its overall objective the construction and maintenance of a social network to prevent the recurrence of a number of social problems (crime and drug and alcohol abuse). The scheme was originally launched as a research project, with the title 'Hyldespjaeldet does something together' and with the intention of drawing in other agencies as well as residents of the project. Financial assistance was received from the research department of the Ministry of Social Affairs.

A number of individual projects were launched, starting in 1989. These were designed to address problems of alcohol abuse and high rates of youth unemployment and provide improved standards of estate management and better community facilities. The evaluation of the project suggests that residents have been successful in launching and managing projects for which they have assumed full responsibility and in providing accessible and popular services. While the experiment was not the responsibility of the municipality, who initially showed little understanding of it, there is now substantial political interest in the outcomes.

Arche Project, Rostock (Germany)

Arche Rostock eV was established in 1991. It is an autonomous non-profit organisation, established to provide employment through construction and rehabilitation projects for use in social programmes. The project is focused upon rehabilitation schemes in severely rundown housing in the old town of Rostock (former East Germany); these schemes are funded mainly from Federal sources, supplied through job-creation schemes for the 'hard-to-place'. The original impetus for the scheme came from an equivalent experiment in Bremen. The intention is to provide a catalyst for co-operation with other agencies and to support networks which will provide assistance for stigmatised and excluded groups. In this capacity, it has received substantial help from the local authority, some of whose staff were heavily but informally involved in setting up the project.

The scheme can be judged a success in terms of achieving the objective of involving stigmatised groups (single parents, 'punks') and providing opportunities for the acquisition of new skills as well as improved housing. As the project has progressed it has acquired more support from official agencies and has become more professional in style; however, the financial base of the project is still not secure.

These projects reflect the very different environment of improvisations with limited resources, with a strong degree of consumer input and some tentative attempts at self-management. They are likely to provide important lessons on the mobilisation of assistance for experimental schemes and the active involvement of user and citizen groups.

Another group of projects make an explicit feature of user 'voice'. The Italian patients' tribunal has grown from the grass roots to gain national coverage and prominence: stressing various aspects of "voice", such as patients' charters, advocacy and quality monitoring, it has extended its activities to direct service provision in some cases. The users' voice is also a feature of the local Wiltshire (UK) community care user involvement network.

Box D   Giving people a voice

Tribunale per i Diritti del Malato (Patient's Rights Tribunal), (Italy)

The TDM is a grass-roots patients' rights movement, part of the broader Movimento Federativo Democratico. Its birth coincided with the reforms creating a national health service, and was designed to protect the principles of equal access to free, high quality, democratically controlled health care by counterbalancing the greater control of political parties and health care professionals. It now has over 400 branches and centres operating in individual hospitals, co-ordinated by regional branches and regional and a national secretariat. It has some public financing, but is largely self-financing and relies mainly on voluntary effort.

Examples of its work include over 70 local patients' charters, a major national survey on the state of patients rights, drafting protective legislation, suggesting and operating local dispute resolution procedures, monitoring the quality of care, advocacy for individuals, local and national protest and lobbying, supporting self-help groups and sometimes directly operating services to fill gaps.

The evaluation suggests that the Tribunale has provided users with an effective instrument to control the production and to a lesser extent the planning of health services. It has also had a powerful influence in promoting dialogue between users and health institutions and users and professional groups (despite early suspicions on the part of the medical profession). There have been improvements in the accessibility, quality and user-friendliness of health care and the initiative is beginning to improve cost-effectiveness.

Community Care User Involvement Network in Wiltshire, (United Kingdom)

The Wiltshire Community Care User Involvement Network started in 1991. It is a user-led independent organisation of people who use the community care services provided by the health, social services and voluntary organisations. It has a membership of older people and people with disabilities, carers and advocates. It was an initiative started by service users and it has now secured funding from the local authority. It aims to overcome the isolation experienced by service users and carers and also to support them in voicing their concerns and working to change staff attitudes and make services more accessible and responsive to users' needs.

The Network has a growing membership and has secured the support of senior managers in the community care services. It has succeeded in empowering its members to become involved in community care strategy development and staff training.

Gender issues have been an important focus for the study, because it is women who form the majority of people in direct contact with the service and women who form the majority of the (usually lower status) staff directly in contact with the public. In most cases, this situation provides an important contextual feature, but in two instances it comes to the fore.

Box E   Women managing change

L'Alliance Project, Issy-les-Moulineaux (France)

L'Alliance is a purpose-built centre established in the middle of Issy, bringing together and actively co-ordinating local services for the domiciliary care of the elderly, both those provided by the municipality and those from the non-profit sector. It was the centrepiece of the municipal plan for provision for the elderly (1991). Although a public sector service, it is intended to provide the focus for a wider collaboration; it is directed towards the improvement of the quality of services and in particular the conditions of the elderly in their homes.

The centre opened in 1993 and at the time of evaluation had only been running for eight months. Nevertheless, substantial gains are reported in the accessibility of services and the quality of the reception given to users calling at the centre. Working conditions for staff and the morale of the team are also reported as being excellent.

Amadora Social Security Office (Portugal)

This service initiative, which was officially launched in 1992, was supported by a central government policy designed to improve the quality of public sector services by increasing social justice and promoting greater equality of opportunity. The Amadora social security office provides a local service co-ordinating the wide range of state, private and independent social security and social welfare agencies. The majority of those using the service are women who come from highly disadvantaged groups. The office is staffed almost entirely by women and the vision and commitment of its two women managers have been important factors in creating and sustaining this service initiative.

The office offers a friendly, popular service which combines respect for citizens with greater efficiency. It has succeeded in bringing the service closer to service users by providing a more accessible, comprehensive and personalised service. It has created valued local job opportunities for women.

The Issy-les-Moulineaux project is also one initiative among several that brought together disparate services in order to provide improved access for users. The Ballyfermot One-Stop Shop (Ireland) is similar - drawing together a range of normally dispersed services and cutting down the pressures on people who use several of them (some of them women with multiple caring responsibilities). Severnside Benefits Agency Office (UK) provides a single service, but with much the same objectives. These two echo the other social security reforms outlined earlier, in that new technology and reformed working arrangements in local offices combine to produce a more user-friendly service.

Box F   Service co-ordination and One-Stop Shops

Ballyfermot One-Stop Shop (Ireland)

The Social Welfare Services Office (SWSO) of the Department of Social Welfare established the Ballyfermot One Stop Shop in a working class suburb of West Dublin, in 1990. The office is purpose built and combines the functions previously discharged in five different locations, mainly in the city centre. These include information on all kinds of benefit, payment of unemployment benefit, processing of new claims and means assessment. The strategic objective of the project is improved customer access to services: increased use of new technology and staff training in client awareness are both features of the project.

The evaluation of the scheme by users was predominantly favourable; and staff considered the office facilities and premises to be of a high standard although there were also problems about the increased level of stressful work. The overall impression is of much improved access to a better integrated service.

Severnside Benefits Agency (UK)

The Severnside District Benefits Agency has taken several initiatives since 1991 to improve the quality of its service for users. The impetus for these initiatives came from the creation of a new national agency - the Benefits Agency - a central government funded organisation delivering social security benefits to citizens. Two of these initiatives - the Community Benefits Council and the Integrated Benefits Counter - were selected for this study. The Community Benefits Council was established to develop a forum for enabling the local community served by the agency to participate in agency development by exchanging views and ideas about the service with agency staff on a regular basis. The Integrated Benefits Counter was opened in 1993 to deliver a range of benefits as well as comprehensive information about benefit eligibility in a new office environment designed with staff advice to improve the physical facilities available to service users.

> During the first six months of its life the Community Benefits Council failed to attract service user representatives. Some representatives from local voluntary organisations involved in advice work began to use the forum to voice their concerns. During the first three months of its life the Integrated Benefits Counter succeeded in dramatically improving the physical service environment for benefit claimants and front line staff. It improved service accessibility for physically disabled service users and for people with reading and writing difficulties. It succeeded in providing a more comprehensive information service to users who have a very positive view of this service change.

The question of access links to that of information: are users aware of the services potentially available to them? In these social security examples there were attempts to break down reticence on both sides of the counter and share information, so as to enable users to gain full access to available benefits.

Two projects are specifically intended to provide new types of facility - in primary health care (Beja, Portugal) and day care of the elderly (KAPI schemes, Greece). In both cases, there is a move away from specialised, professionally dominated institutional services, in favour of building a team which relates more closely to the everyday lives of ordinary people. And in both cases the charismatic leadership of non-conformist professionals was vital, but in very different circumstances. In Portugal, change was achieved in spite of dominant policies and regulations; in Greece there was a happy marriage between these new ideas and broader political imperatives.

Box G   Extending the range of services

Beja Regional Health Centre (Portugal)

The Beja region is one of the most underprivileged regions of Portugal. This initiative was officially launched in the Aljustrel Health Centre in 1988. It was designed to improve the primary health care provided for citizens in this region. It used a model of primary health care developed by the World Health Organisation. This model replaced the existing hierarchical, medically dominated specialist primary health teams with multidisciplinary primary health care teams collectively responsible for managing primary health care resources and their delivery to designated catchment areas. The success of this initiative in Aljustrel has led to its adoption in other parts of the region, and subsequently in other regions.

Evidence of the success of this initiative can be found in the way in which it increased the numbers of citizens accessing primary health care in the region, the continuity of professional contact it delivered to users and the marked improvements in maternity and post natal infant care it provided. Staff involved reported increased job satisfaction and noted an increase in the coverage as well as the quality of their work.

Open Care Old People's Centres (Kapis), (Greece)

Kapis were initially introduced in Greece on a small scale in the late 1970s and expanded throughout the country in the 1980s. They are part of a 'stay-at-home' policy for old people and provide a wide range of professional services - social work, occupational therapy, physiotherapy and leisure facilities. The concept is a new departure for Greece and stems originally from a single-handed campaign by an official of the Ministry of Health, Welfare and Social Security, which eventually linked with the overall programme of decentralisation introduced by the Socialist government. The involvement of local government followed and has been crucial to the success of the projects. The four Kapis in Nea Ionia are largely the creation of an individual politician, the Communist mayor, although they were likewise supported elsewhere by local mayors.

The Kapis are innovative not just in the character of the service they provide but also in introducing the notion of a meeting place based on membership, where members participate actively and form part of the management committee. The evaluation suggests that Kapis have provided greatly improved access to services which used to be either inaccessible or too expensive. Staff were also generally in favour of the overall concept and accepting of the greatly enhanced role played by users in deciding the ways in which the services are organised and delivered. Inevitably there were divisions between staff, users and local authorities over some issues, such as funding.

A final central theme of the work programme has been the effect on the staff of new initiatives that are designed to improve the quality of services for users. Two contrasting studies, one in France and one in Denmark, show some of the consequences for staff of the ways in which new initiatives have been introduced. The second study is particularly helpful in illustrating comparatively some of the consequences of ways in which resources have been allocated.

Box H   Local experiments in different methods of service delivery

Office Municipal d'HLM Nantes-Habitat (France)

This project is based on the reforms introduced into the public housing sector (HLMs) of Nantes after the election of a new (Socialist) Mayor in March 1989. The Mayor also holds the office of president of the administrative council of the Office Municipal d'HLMs and has used this to introduce major structural changes into the management and delivery of the municipal housing service. The objectives of these reforms, carried out by a new director, were to bring the service closer to the tenants by introducing a system of decentralised offices, improving the quality of service offered by providing better information and a more welcoming reception service, improved financial management and repairs and rehabilitation of the housing stock. All this was in the context of the 'social mission' of the agency and involved a substantial investment in the retraining of staff.

The evaluation suggests that there has been a substantial improvement in accessibility and housing quality. The staff, too, are conscious of substantial improvements in their working conditions - this is reflected in improved morale. The role of the mayor in providing continuity of political support has been important for the long-term success of the project.

Integrated Care Service for the Elderly, Odense (Denmark)

In November 1989, Odense Municipality started an experimental scheme designed to provide a 24-hour care service for the elderly. This covered both pre-arranged visits and emergency cover. The use of radio technology makes it possible to maintain reliable communication between a base and the individual home help or nurse on duty. The service was intended to replace previous separate provision divided between nursing homes and home helps working with old people in the community. The specific objectives of the scheme were to facilitate a more flexible deployment of staff and create as far as possible a unified service for all old people, regardless of whether they lived in an institution or their own home. The scheme integrated all the services and provided for close collaboration between all categories of staff, working in groups.

The evaluation of the experiment found that the public were generally critical of the new system but that this was largely because the Odense municipality made cuts in the resources available during the course of the experiment: the public were particularly concerned that the new service did not appear to be reliable. The staff, who had been entrusted with greater responsibility as members of the semi-autonomous groups sharing the jobs of planning and allocation of work, also found the transition difficult. However, there was a sharp contrast in experience between the two sub-areas in which the experimental scheme had been introduced - both staff changes and budget cuts impacted far more heavily in one area and this crucially affected staff and user satisfaction.

Summary and Conclusions

This chapter has summarised the evidence from the sixteen local case studies. The description of the national and local case studies is now complete; in the next three chapters the significance of the detailed findings from the research will be assessed.

CHAPTER FIVE :   Aims and Achievements

The projects represent variations on a number of similar themes established in a range of national contexts and were certainly not conceived as part of a coherent EU-wide programme of action. In order to highlight similarities and differences, then, this chapter begins by providing a summary of the targets for the projects, delineating particular aspects of the consumer orientation and then noting associated objectives.

The second part of the chapter introduces the questions against which the European Foundation asked researchers to evaluate each project. It goes on to summarise the answers to some of those questions - those concerned with an overall evaluation. The responses to questions specifically concerned with equal opportunities are incorporated into the following chapter. The discussion of the results of the case studies is completed by a commentary on the process of change.

Before any substantial analysis can take place, however, some preliminary remarks are necessary, first about the basis of the evaluations and then about the nature of the services involved.

The Problem of Evaluation

Many of the projects described here are major initiatives, upon which significant resources of money, time and effort, and often great human concern have been invested. It is surprising, therefore that in only a few instances were clear (let alone measurable) targets for improvement identified in advance - especially in those instances where the changes were imposed from the top downwards. It is, similarly, surprising that evaluations of the process and outcomes of change were not more frequent. Indeed, in some instances even basic monitoring data were limited.

Thus, the evaluations done as a result of this project quite often represented the only formal review of the initiatives and their outcomes. On occasion, too, the evaluators were confronted with limited information on which to base their judgements and these gaps had to be filled by retrospective investigation and analysis.

Evidently, the process of evaluation is often neither easy nor uncontentious. Different interested parties can come to very different conclusions, so that evaluations must often be pluralistic, especially if lessons are to be learned about the process of change; so the Foundation research sought to capture the perspectives of managers, staff and users. Furthermore, any new initiative is often the child of earlier ones and the parent of others, while yet more changes interact with it, so that it becomes impossible to set finite boundaries around the initiative or its impacts. This is especially the case in those changes which were not initiated from the top and were more concerned with starting out in a particular direction than arriving at a pre-conceived destination. One element in this equation was the nature of the service itself.

Cash and Kind

Six of the services entailed the distribution of money; nine were concerned with services in kind, such as health, social care and housing; one contained a mix of cash and social welfare services.

Cash services emanate from well-established bureaucracies. Even if they began as mutual aid organisations, it has been thought necessary, for reasons of equity, efficiency and social solidarity, for these bodies to be large in scale and to operate according to strict rules of entitlement (for pensions), or tightly regulated discretion (for social security). Where it exists, consumer involvement is of a representative nature, distanced from the individual. Interactions between staff and users are limited in scope and concern the application of those rules. In these circumstances it is easy for the rules and the internal operation of the organisation to dominate, at the expense of consumer interests.

Opportunities for consumer involvement in any changes are also likely to be limited: they may entail some consultation about the options for change - and in all our cases these changes concerned methods of service delivery rather than entitlements - and then an emphasis on access, information and redress as a consequence of any reform. There are limitations, too, upon staff involvement at the planning stage. Common organisational patterns encompassing many offices are likely to be necessary, so involvement is initially probably through representative mechanisms. Widespread staff participation during the implementation stage is unlikely - unless there is a local demonstration project first.

Services in kind are often markedly different. Locally varying patterns of organisation may obtain; and staff - especially professional staff - have scope to innovate and to adapt both the content and delivery of services. Such scope has sometimes led to the pursuance of provider interests or to the elaboration of specialisms which have the effect of making services less accessible to the customer. On the other hand, the active participation of consumers is often needed for the service to be delivered successfully, so that there is an element of co-production. As a result a wide range of mechanisms of participation is potentially available to staff and users alike.

Consumer Orientations and Associated Ends and Means

Tables 5.1 and 5.2 summarise the precise aspects of consumer orientation which were sought in the various change initiatives and the other features which accompanied or enabled it.

Improved **quality** of service, which included improvements to the physical environment, the friendliness with which people are received, responsiveness to their needs and speedier services, was a universal aim. This was often linked to improved access - most commonly localisation, but also access for people with physical or sensory impairments (the general question of equal opportunities will be discussed in Chapter 6).

The **integration** of previously disparate services was another common feature, closely associated with responsiveness and access. The common aim was to limit the number of people or places it was necessary to visit in order to gain access to the services needed. In the case of financial payments this was mostly through more generic staff roles (although the range of benefits available might still be narrow). It was more likely to be through multi-disciplinary or inter-disciplinary working (or perhaps simply the common location of several specialists) in the case of services in kind.

Improved access to **information** was also attempted in several cases, whether for services in cash or kind. Like other aims this could be seen as part of a package of measures to treat people as consumers, entitled to convenient services of a high standard. To take market-style consumerism to its logical conclusion also implies powers of **choice and exit**. The relevance of such concepts for public services is a matter of controversy. Some argue that the proper exercise of choice is through the political process and that, in any case, choice at the point of entry gives limited power in respect of complex and slowly maturing goods, like pensions, or experiential goods such as social care. Others claim that the power to take one's custom elsewhere would transform relations in public services. Be that as it may, none of the initiatives in this study offered any choice between service providers and in only two instances was choice between different services within the same agency a minor feature.

In public services, the traditional alternative to choice is **voice** - implying a more active involvement in decisions about what services to provide and how to deliver them. This can only be relatively modest at the point where people receive cash services, since key decisions have been made earlier and elsewhere. Our cases include some collective involvement in planning and monitoring service delivery in Bremen (Prosoz) and the Severnside benefits office (UK) and an individual one in staff-consumer interactions (Italy: Pensione Subito). The expression of voice was more common and more successful with respect to services in kind: indeed it was the major feature of Italian health tribunals and the Wiltshire Community Care User Involvement Network. Active **participation** in the planning and delivery of services also characterised several of the health, social care and social action developments e.g. Beja health centre, Portugal, and this was extended to self-management and control in Italy (Tribunals), Denmark (Social Network) and, in a more uncertain way, to Rostock (Arche). Measures for increased **accountability** or for redress were, however, less in evidence.

TABLE 5.1   Which aspects of consumer orientation?

	Cash services										Services in kind					
	Pensione Subito	IKA Pensions	Prosoz	QUIP	Severnside	Ballyfermot	Amadora	Tribunale	Beja Health	Kapi	Odense	L'Alliance	Wiltshire	Nantes Habitat	Rostock Arche	Hyldesp jaeldet
Information	**			*	**	**	**	**	*			**	**	**		
Access	**	**	**		**	**	**	**	**	**	*	**	**	**		
Service integration	*		**		**	**	**		**	**	*	**			**	**
Quality · responsiveness · speed, better facilities	**	**	**	**	**	**	**	**	**	**	**	**	**	**	**	**
Voice	*		*		*			**	*	**			**		**	**
Participation								*	*	**			**		**	**
Choice										*						*
Redress								**								
Accountability								**						*		
Self management & control by users								**	*	*					*	**

Key :   ** =   major element
        * =   contributory element of more limited importance or scope

61

As Table 5.2 indicates, **managerial reform** was a universal feature as regards cash services, albeit to varying degrees. This was often linked to wider structural reform in which senior managers were given greater freedom, and would be judged according to their achievements. Often the means chosen to achieve such changes were a combination of information technology and forms of job enlargement which gave greater discretion to local staff, especially those at the front line. Fewer levels of management might also result.

Managerialist reforms were much less in evidence for services in kind and their impacts here were less uniform: in Wiltshire they were tied in with a stronger expression of consumer voice; in Italy, those voices were raised as a reaction against managerialist centralisation.

The approach to **technological change** also contrasted sharply: most of the new technologies employed for caring services were of an intermediate kind - a retreat from technical specialisms towards closer links with natural helping networks and remedies. The shift to integrated primary health care and indigenous treatments in Beja, and to community care in Nea Ionia, Issy and Wiltshire are cases in point. In Nea Ionia, for example, old people were less likely to be cast as patients in institutions and more as members of community-based clubs - posing a challenge for staff attitudes and work patterns. In Amadora, the pattern of work of the office was changed to fit the rhythm of the lives of women consumers and workers. Even in Odense, where radio communication was introduced, it was linked to self-managing groups of community health care staff.

Despite these differences in chosen means however, an improvement in **organisational efficiency** was a common aim across the case studies, if not a primary one. This was sometimes linked to **cost containment**, but in this respect the motivations and consequences were more complex. For services in kind, where the initiatives were often local, the scarcity of resources was seen as more of a constraint to be lived with or overcome, rather than an overt aim. And in some instances it was a distinct threat to the success of the initiative as changes were begun, only to be held back as a result of

TABLE 5.2   Associated ends and means

	Cash services								Services in kind							
	Pensione Subito	IKA Pensions	Prosoz	QUIP	Severnside	Ballyfermot	Amadora	Tribunale	Beja Health	Kapi	Odense	L'Alliance	Wiltshire	Nantes Habitat	Rostock Arche	Hyldespj aeldet
Cost containment	*		*	T				*R	C	C	T		C		C	
Organisational efficiency	**	**	**	*	*			*	*		*	**		**		
Managerialism	**	*	**	**	*	*	*	R				*	**	**		
Decentralisation	**	*	**	*	*	*	*		*		**	*				
New technology	**	**	**	*	**	**	*		I	I	*		I	*	I	I

Key :

**	=	major element or aim
*	=	contributory elements or aim
T	=	threat to the success of the initiative
C	=	constraint within which initiative took place
R	=	initiative represents a reaction against dangers of such moves
I	=	intermediate technology stressing self-help and social networks

stringency. The Italian health case is even more paradoxical, since it contains examples of campaigns against cuts and closures, as well as wars on waste to mitigate their effects.

Evaluative Questions

In order to provide a common basis for judging the achievements of the project, evaluators sought evidence on a range of topics. These concerned:

* user involvement in the planning of services
* user involvement in the provision of services
* improvements in service quality
* improvements in working conditions
* other intended consequences
* impact on costs
* unintended consequences.

Questions were asked about two further matters: improvements in both the quality of services and working conditions for women in particular; and the political support for and later diffusion of the initiatives. These will be addressed in Chapters 6 and 7 respectively. It is important to stress that these questions have been posed after the event. In what follows, the intention is not to criticise people for failing to achieve outcomes to which they never aspired, but rather to make clear when any particular objective was assessed. Similarly, it must be borne in mind that both relative priority given to these various objectives and also the precise way in which they were framed varied considerably, while limitations on the data available will have reduced both the precision and scope of the findings. Nonetheless, the national reports unveiled a wealth of evaluative material, which is summarised below.

Overview of Impacts

User involvement

There were relatively few cases in which user involvement in planning was aimed for, and several of these had limited success. In those where it featured strongly - the Wiltshire

Community Care Network, the Italian Patients' Tribunals, the Hyldespjaeldet Social Network and, to a more mixed extent, the Rostock Arche - there was a strong emphasis upon self-organisation of users, based on a common identity. It is not surprising that two of these entailed the self-management of services. Where services were being provided by the statutory authority, user involvement in planning led to demands for significant change, going beyond the providers' agenda, and involvement in provision and management by users remained an option (Wiltshire Community Care, Patients' Tribunals).

User involvement in service provision was rather more common, although it remained modest and tightly linked to the providers' agenda in respect of cash services. Here, the setting of explicit service standards was sometimes seen as a means of enhancing consumer power and this was borne out in Severnside UK. It also applied in the Health Tribunals. More usually, however, consumer power in the provision of services in kind depended on, and led to, stronger calls for a more holistic approach in which professionals, sharing power, took greater account of the fact that users did not experience services singly but in combination with other services and in the context of their daily lives (Wiltshire Community Care, Kapi Centres Greece, Amadora and Beja Health, Portugal). Of course self-management in Hyldespjaeldet and some Rostock Arche services provide the extreme examples of people's empowerment.

TABLE 5.3	User involvement in planning	User involvement in service provision
Pensione Subito, Italy	None.	Staff and consumers shared the task of calculating pension entitlements. People were informed/reminded of the existence of various advisory and advocacy agencies and made more use of them. There is a danger however that user power will suffer if the role of these agencies is usurped.

TABLE 5.3 (contd.)	User involvement in planning	User involvement in service provision
IKA Pensions, Greece	None.	None.
Prosoz Bremen, Germany	Consumers participated in the steering group, but had little influence, except in minor issues.	Requests for information about criteria used and administrative processes were refused: users remain supplicants.
QUIP, Ireland	Some consumer opinion surveys, but otherwise not involved.	None.
Severnside Benefits Office, UK	Attempts to involve consumers in an advisory group failed.	Better access, published performance standards and complaints all led to greater consumer influence.
Ballyfermot One-Stop Shop, Ireland	Significant user consultation.	None.
Amadora Social Security, Portugal	None: information and participation are lacking.	None: stronger guarantees of service standards, more regular opinion surveys, more mediating bodies and consumer education are needed.
Patients' Rights Tribunals, Italy	Some local societies have become heavily involved in planning health care: they focus on the enforcement of existing laws and standards to protect consumers. The impact is variable and hard to measure, overall.	The strong focus on the enforcement of existing rules and standards to protect patients, and the negotiation of new ones, has given consumers real power - but it varies locally and the overall impact is hard to measure.

TABLE 5.3 (contd.)	User involvement in planning	User involvement in service provision
Beja Health, Portugal	The model adopted implies community involvement in health planning, but there is some way to go to make this effective.	The holistic approach to people's health, which analyses health needs in context and by age group, not disease category, allows greater influence over the care which is provided.
Kapi Centres for Older People, Greece	Not prior to initial establishment.	Members have their own local committee, which elects representatives onto the Kapi management board, as well as exercising informal influence. Their influence has surprised many and has led to a greater emphasis on recreational services.
Odense integrated care for elderly people, Denmark	There has been no direct influence, although planning now takes place closer to the customer.	Needs-based principles have been adopted in the nursing homes, but general regulations and design constraints have limited their impact. Community users may now have less influence, due to supply problems and the use of staff from the nursing homes, who have an institutional orientation.
Alliance Older People's Centre, France	None.	More user-responsive services may lead to a modest rise in influence, but the group lacks political identity and power.

TABLE 5.3 (contd.)	User involvement in planning	User involvement in service provision
Wiltshire Community Care Users' Network, UK	This was a major and successful focus, based on organised groups with a planning remit. Resources to enable user self-organisation were crucial. When user defined, community care was as much about citizenship and equal access to mainstream life as it was about service provision, and the local state needed to support such equal participation as citizens.	Services which are seen as relevant to users' own definition of needs may emerge from this process, but it is too soon to judge. They are likely to go beyond social care services, cutting across existing organisational boundaries and challenging dominant assumptions about disability.
Habitat, Nantes, France	Never an objective: representation is too weak at this level.	Practically nil: consultations had little influence on decisions. However, the high political profile meant that reactions expressed through the media might cause speedy modifications.
Rostock Arche, Germany	Users of accommodation schemes had considerable influence over the initial definition of needs and how they might be met. Those involved in employment and job training had no influence.	Users of accommodation and similar services would have a heavy involvement in the management of services when completed. Those on employment and training schemes had little influence, but their main concerns were about quality.

TABLE 5.3 (contd.)	User involvement in planning	User involvement in service provision
Hyldespjaeldet Social Network Project, Denmark	There was complete control of planning for the project.	Full control of management and implementation, including the employment of staff. This did, however, lead to disputes over the discretion taken by informal project leaders.

Information and access

Improved information and access were much more ubiquitous aims, being the major targets in many instances. It is in these respects, too, that the highest rate of success was achieved. Decentralisation and service integration markedly increased consumer satisfaction with the convenience of services and frequently led to greater demand which could be satisfied more economically and efficiently. In addition, access to new forms of service was provided in many instances.

TABLE 5.4	Information and access
Pensione Subito, Italy	Information about services provided by the scheme and about independent advisory bodies was improved. Localised offices in which one member of staff dealt with all aspects of a person's claim greatly enhanced access for personal callers, who also enjoyed better reception areas. The general public continued to criticise access by telephone, despite efforts to improve it.
IKA Pensions, Greece	People were enabled to call at localised offices, which could handle all aspects of pensions work and had discretion to take decisions.
Prosoz Social Security, Germany	Decentralised, integrated offices gave people easier access to all aspects of their claim for benefits.
QUIP, Ireland	There were improvements in office facilities for the public, certificates could be registered locally and the response to telephone enquiries improved.

TABLE 5.4 (contd.)	Information and access
Severnside Benefits Office, UK	Benefits 'surgeries' were held in local communities. Physical access to the new local office was made much easier, while the Integrated Benefits Counter reduced social barriers to access, especially for people with reading and writing difficulties. More comprehensive information was also provided.
Ballyfermot One-Stop Shop, Ireland	There was a very high level of awareness of the new locally integrated service, which provided very significantly improved access and reduced travel and time costs. There were very heavy demands made for information on a wide range of issues, although the limited information available about job opportunities could be further extended. Access for voluntary and welfare workers who acted as advocates was also increased. Consumers also report considerable gains in the social accessibility of a more user-friendly service.
Amadora Social Security, Portugal	Decentralised offices and improved facilities, along with better personal, written and telephone contacts all led to a significant improvement in access. A survey of users indicated that they valued the physical environment, the friendly reception from staff and the information provided by the office.
Patients' Rights Tribunals, Italy	In some areas gaps in the locally available services were filled; mothers' access to their hospitalised children improved and outpatient appointments were speeded up.
Beja Health, Portugal	There has been a significant increase in the coverage of primary health care services and consumers can and do make use of them at an earlier stage, so that potential problems can be prevented or detected sooner.
Kapi Centres for Older People, Greece	There have been major gains in access: services which were unavailable, or difficult and expensive to reach, are now found at local level and altogether Kapis have 65,000 members.

TABLE 5.4 (contd.)	Information and access
Integrated care for elderly people, Odense, Denmark	Access to services is still through professional assessment of need and targeting services towards the "most needy" reduced access for some people. However, the services are now more generic, once people have gained entry to them.
Alliance Elderly People's Centre, France	Co-ordinated services provided from an accessible central point have improved access to diverse systems of help. The friendly and speedy reception facilities also reduce social barriers. Access to those services provided in people's own homes has not changed, but users have benefitted from improved co-ordination of services.
Wiltshire Community Care Users' Network, UK	There has as yet been no attempt to improve physical access. Services should become more socially accessible as providers cease those practices which lead to users being disempowered.
Habitat, Nantes, France	Physical access has greatly increased now that the offices are decentralised. They have also become more socially accessible, as the inner workings of the bureaucracy have been de-mystified and staff have learned more about the problems faced by tenants. More information is also on hand.
Rostock Arche, Germany	By converting buildings so that various community projects can use them, Arche is giving access to services for excluded minorities which, otherwise, would not be available.
Hyldespjaeldet Social Network, Denmark	Services were aimed at a wide range of people and attempts to include all of those needing particular services were mostly successful. Since services were provided on the estate - mostly in people's own homes - they were very accessible.

Service Quality

Improvements to information and access were closely linked to the question of service quality. Relations with staff were also high on the agenda for change. Thus in all cash-based services, except the Greek case, significant improvements were reported in such matters as speedier payment, reduced queues and waiting times, better facilities while waiting and a friendlier reception by staff who were more responsive to people's needs. Quality improvements for services in kind often require a longer period of maturation before they become evident and in several instances (eg Rostock, Wiltshire and Odense) it was too soon for considered judgements to be made. In both our health care cases, however, significant gains were reported, while the two centres for older people also contributed to an improved quality of life for their users.

TABLE 5.5	Service quality
Pensione Subito, Italy	The time spent waiting to receive a pension was significantly reduced, there were shorter queues at the office and the quality of relationships between users and staff improved. Other aspects, such as the procedure for determining entitlements, were not part of the project, and remained problematic.
IKA Pensions, Greece	Limited evaluative data were collected, but there appeared to be modest improvements. However, shortage of skilled staff and of space, and the neglect of complementary improvements in work organisation and computer facilities limited the impact.
Prosoz Social Security Payments, Bremen, Germany	There were gains in the speed, reliability, responsiveness and flexibility of services, within the boundaries of essentially bureaucratic procedures.
QUIP, Ireland	Application forms were simplified, the response to claims speeded up, as were payment procedures. People received a fuller and quicker answer to queries, while signposting, privacy and comfort also improved.
Severnside Benefits Office, UK	The integrated benefits counter led to a dramatic improvement in the quality of service for consumers, whose views on the change were very positive.
Ballyfermot One-Stop Shop, Ireland	People liked the friendly service, its continuity from one member of staff and the improvements in comfort and privacy. A range of services were now available in one place, and they were better integrated. Power relations were unchanged.

TABLE 5.5 (contd.)	Service quality
Amadora Social Security, Portugal	Levels of public satisfaction were influenced by ignorance about the internal changes and were neither very high nor very low on a range of indicators. However, the evaluators spoke of appreciable improvements in co-ordination between services and in consumer-centredness. More significant improvements would be dependent upon larger budgets, improved training and management capacity, information technology and clearer performance and service standards.
Patients' Rights Tribunal, Italy	In some localities, and for some groups of users, such as women with sick children, profound increases in quality have occurred, but local variation, the wide scope of the movement and its complex ramifications make accurate measurement impossible. In general, people are more conscious of their health and of their rights, and working practices and staff attitudes have improved.
Beja Health, Portugal	Over 5 years there has been a 12.5% increase in medical care, with better coverage of the population, earlier intervention and greater continuity. Infant mortality has declined. Care has become more personalised and bureaucratic procedures reduced. The general crisis in health care, lack of resources and the effects of inappropriate centralised rules and policies have limited the potential improvements, however.
Kapi Centres for Older People, Greece	This is a new service which has led to dramatic improvements for people able to use the centres. These include a reduction in power differentials which normally obtain between users and professionals, so that services are shaped to people's preferences.
Integrated Care, Odense, Denmark	In the short term many people experienced a deterioration of services due to difficulties in planning to meet conflicting demands from the nursing homes and community, exacerbated by financial restrictions in one area. Reliability of service suffered. The hope is that these transitional problems will decrease and integration will enable services to tailor-make their provision to individual needs.

TABLE 5.5 (contd.)	Service quality
Alliance Older People's Centre, France	The environment was much more welcoming and user-friendly: users remarked that staff took the time and interest to listen. They could also respond in a more coherent fashion since staff from various disciplines came together into a team surprisingly quickly. The range of available services has expanded. Previously hidden needs of older people and their carers became evident, however, planting the seeds of further change.
Wiltshire Community Care Network, UK	Professionals believe that services have improved considerably, but they started from a very low baseline. The increased voice (not power) of consumers is expected to feed through into more significant service improvements and more acceptable services in due course.
Habitat, Nantes, France	The initiative met its objectives of providing a speedier, more acceptable and user friendly response to tenants' concerns. Shortage of accommodation remains one of the major problems.
Rostock Arche, Germany	The quality of training and support for people on employment schemes suffered, due to lack of permanent staff, although matters were improving as resources were made available. Most of the accommodation schemes were not yet in operation when the evaluation took place, but they offered the hope of significant improvement.
Hyldespjaeldet Social Network, Denmark	The services provided were very adaptable to local people's needs and circumstances.

Working conditions for staff

The impact of the changes upon the working conditions for staff was rather more mixed. Most staff appreciated the shorter journeys which came from localised services, and, indeed, the local availability of work itself. They also enjoyed the improved environment, not only for its physical comfort, but also how it led to better relations between themselves and users and to pride in providing higher quality services. Such improved quality also came from the changes in working practices which enabled them as individuals to deal with most of a consumer's needs, rather than being an anonymous element of a fragmented process. Those changes gave many staff richer and more responsible jobs.

The other side of the coin was that the demands upon staff increased. Closer and more extensive and open contact with consumers was one element of this - in the form of sustained criticism and pressure to change services in the Italian Health Tribunals and in Wiltshire, and of some intimidation when rules and rationing criteria were applied in Severnside, Ballyfermot and Nantes. Equally the content of the work and the performance standards expected became more exacting. Adequate training and equipment, supportive procedures and management and remuneration which matched greater effort were widely seen as the ways to balance these increased responsibilities and pressures.

Of these needs, training and equipment were the most likely to be provided: this was the case in nearly all of the social security and pensions reforms - the exceptions being Amadora and IKA Pensions, Greece; it was less in evidence in relation to other services, where the changes were less predictable and demanded perhaps significant adaptation and self-discovery over time. There also needed to be greater recognition that multi-disciplinary working needed to be managed, with senior management processes supporting and rewarding it (Beja Health, Greek Kapis, Odense Integrated Care). Indeed, some difficulties with the requisite changes in management - moving from specialised hierarchical command and control through layers of management, to supporting, guiding and enabling front-line discretion from a strategic core - were noted in several cases (Italy Pensions, QUIP Ireland, Amadora Social Security and Beja Health Portugal, and Odense Integrated Care Denmark). Lastly, in few cases was increased responsibility matched by increased financial rewards for front-line staff.

TABLE 5.6	Improving working conditions
Pensione Subito, Italy	New technology and decentralised responsibility led to increased skills, bigger jobs and a greater valuing of front-line staff. On the other hand, pressure to work quickly and to higher standards increased, so that jobs became more arduous: there was limited recognition of this and of the importance and difficulty of working close to the consumers, who also expected staff to help in their relations with less accessible sections. Promotion prospects were also limited.
IKA Pensions, Greece	Some staff moving to de-centralised offices benefited from enriched jobs and higher status, but these benefits were restricted by poor facilities and insufficient training. Those who were obliged to move to staff decentralised functions were inconvenienced.
Prosoz Social Security Payments, Bremen, Germany	Staff were heavily involved in the process of change, which achieved widespread acceptance. The work of front-line staff was enriched and it became easier to process cases. However, staff shortages and rationalisation plans brought problems and hostility.
QUIP, Ireland	New technology has led to less manual work and the development of better working practices. Staff involved in the quality teams enjoyed the opportunities to develop their skills and to work as teams, so that their self-esteem rose. However, they lacked any tangible reward for their efforts, were frustrated by the slow response by managers to their proposals and experienced an anti-climax when they returned to ordinary work. Several went elsewhere for promotion.
Severnside Benefits Office, UK	Physical conditions for work were much improved and the integrated benefits counter enabled staff to have much better relations with consumers, and greater job satisfaction. They were, however, concerned about the risk of violence.

TABLE 5.6 (contd.)	Improving working conditions
Ballyfermot One-Stop Shop, Ireland	Staff enjoyed working in localised offices, closer to home; they appreciated the improved both physical environment and the access to new technology, for themselves and for the improved service it offered to consumers. There was also some increase in promotion prospects. However increased demands, and pressure from some consumers which occasionally led to threats were a cause of concern.
Amadora Social Security, Portugal	Staff appreciated the opportunity to work locally, rather than having to commute to Lisbon, and also the improved working environment and access to other staff. There were limited opportunities for training, however.
Patients' Rights Tribunals, Italy	The initiative was not aimed at staff, but it has had a strong, but variable and incalculable impact upon both their work and their outlook upon it.
Beja Health, Portugal	Simplified procedures, greater discretion and multi-disciplinary working have led to improvements. These are limited by lack of training, a shortage of specialist staff and other resources, and centralised rules, one of which rewards vertical career paths, rather than co-ordinated working.
Kapi Older People's Centres, Greece	These were new services, so that comparison with the past is difficult. The lack of a clear management process led to self-determination among staff and some inter-professional rivalry.
Odense Integrated Care, Denmark	Most found the move to self-managing teams covering both residential and community services difficult to cope with. These problems were exacerbated by staff reductions in one locality, so that the overall impact was judged to be negative. Extra demands to provide relief cover were especially burdensome and there was a significant turn-over of staff.
Alliance Older People's Centre, France	Staff from the various services were generally pleased to work together in a pleasant and welcoming environment which was near to the town's social and administrative facilities. Working relations were much improved and team work was quickly established.

TABLE 5.6 (contd.)	Improving working conditions
Wiltshire Community Care Network, UK	The initiative has made life more difficult for staff, as they have struggled to adapt to more confident, knowledgeable and powerful users.
Habitat, Nantes, France	Decentralisation has provided better physical working conditions, in which the work has become more interesting and staff have been freer to manage it and work together as a team. They have developed a strong positive image of themselves and the service they provide. However the increased work which arises from the decentralisation has not been matched by increased remuneration.
Rostock Arche, Germany	People have gained work experience - and some have jobs - where none existed before. In other respects no clear conclusions can be drawn.
Hyldespjaeldet Social Network, Denmark	The work was relevant, meaningful and satisfying, but also demanded greater flexibility and commitment. Job security was poor.

Impact on costs

It was noted earlier that there was considerable variation in the stance taken to various forms of cost. On the one hand, it was recognised that new services had to be resourced, as did improvements in physical conditions. On the other, improvements in cost-effectiveness were definite targets in some reforms, while financial constraint was a constant theme, sometimes at the heart of the objectives and sometimes creating crises which cut across the achievement of planned objectives (Odense Integrated Care, Greek Pensions and Old People Centres, QUIP Ireland, Prosoz Germany). There were measurable improvements in cost-effectiveness in the Prosoz scheme and indications that improved services were being provided with more or less the same operating resources in Habitat France, Beja Portugal and the Irish QUIP scheme.

TABLE 5.7	Impact on costs
Pensione Subito, Italy	No data
IKA Pensions, Greece	Not a consideration and no data.
Prosoz Social Security Payments, Bremen, Germany	Large savings in operating costs due to 25% increase in speed of case - processing and a reduction of unproductive other work. Direct costs of the change met by Federal Ministry of Research and Technology. Later rationalisation thwarted some planned changes.
QUIP, Ireland	Not an objective, but an annual saving of IR£22,300 was noted.
Severnside Benefits Office, UK	Almost £1/2M was spent on capital improvement. No record of impact on operating costs.
Ballyfermot One-Stop Shop, Ireland	Increased considerably in the short-term. There is hope for savings in the longer term, due to higher productivity and less fraud and overpayment.
Amadora Social Security, Portugal	No data.
Patients' Rights Tribunals, Italy	Not possible to estimate: some state subsidy. Various campaigns to increase efficiency and also to protect services from closure.
Beja Health, Portugal	No data.
Kapi Older People's Centres, Greece	New service, leading to public expenditure, but possible savings elsewhere. Shift of financial responsibility from centre to locality threatened their future, not least because they had been more generously funded than local services.
Odense Integrated Care, Denmark	Normal expectation was for a neutral impact on costs, or a slight decrease. In fact, one locality had a slight rise in staff, the other was cut back due to general financial stringency.
Alliance Older People's Centre, France	Cost containment not an objective: extra costs needed to open and run the centre.
Wiltshire Community Care Network, UK	Increased costs to fund network found by switching resources at a time of financial stringency.

TABLE 5.7 (contd.)	Impacts on costs
Habitat, Nantes, France	No data: extra costs are presumed to have been balanced by increased efficiency. Budgets must balance, and any increase in rents would have to be justified.
Rostock Arche, Germany	Arche attracts Federal and European funds to provide these new services. There has been some indirect local funding in the form of staff time.
Hyldespjaeldet Social Network, Denmark	Initially, a small special grant was used. Now financed through unorthodox use of traditional subsidies. Voluntary effort is a significant element.

Other impacts

The other changes noted by evaluators mainly concerned increased demand - for new services (Alliance France, Ballyfermot Ireland), for different sorts of service (Kapi Greece and especially Wiltshire UK) and for more of existing services. In short, giving power and influence to consumers can be unpredictable and uncomfortable and demands a partnership with staff who are used to control. It will also (as in Hyldespjaeldet) require more explicit guidelines to protect the basic rights of both minority users and staff.

TABLE 5.8	Other impacts [1]
IKA Pensions, Greece	Minor variation in interpretation of standard rules about pension entitlements.
Prosoz, Bremen, Germany	Improved skills of case processors.
Severnside Benefits Office, UK	Consultation with users not as effective as hoped. Improved access and quality may lead to increased demand at a time when government is attempting to contain it.

---

1. Where none were noted, the project has been omitted.

TABLE 5.8 (contd.)	Other impacts
Ballyfermot One-Stop Shop, Ireland	Increased demand for information led to demands for more staff. Localised staffing led to increased intimidation of staff.
Kapi Older People's Centres, Greece	The strength of consumer influence and the emphasis on leisure services were not anticipated.
Alliance Older People's Centre, France	Unexpectedly high demands for supportive information systems, management and staff support. Discovery of the needs of informal carers led to further enlargement of the team.
Wiltshire Community Care Network, UK	As intended, the influence of users over professionals has grown, but there is a danger that they will be absorbed, within the existing system, rather than challenging it.
Habitat, Nantes, France	Some measures towards consumers were resisted by staff, who saw them as increasing managerial supervision. Staff exposed to violence, being closer to the consumer.
Rostock Arche, Germany	The project became an intermediary between official bodies and informal initiatives among hard-to-reach groups.
Hyldespjaeldet Social Network, Denmark	Local discretion and self-management had the effect of increasing access for some and decreasing it for others. Delegation needs to be within standard guidelines to protect vulnerable groups.

Summary and Conclusions

Many of the changes described have been successful in combatting exclusion by ensuring that disadvantaged people are given better access to an improved quality of basic services, which reflect their dignity as human beings, rather than demeaning it. Some have also extended the availability of specific supportive services to vulnerable groups who previously lacked them. Staff have shared in these improvements, both for themselves and for the satisfaction of providing services of which they could feel proud.

While they have had support in this process, however, they have shouldered a good deal of the responsibility for these improvements themselves, and with limited recognition of this fact. In only two cases (Rostock Arche and Hyldespjaeldet) was it a major objective to assist disadvantaged groups to move from the margin to the mainstream by providing a route to occupational skills and employment. Such a challenge was looming elsewhere (Wiltshire, in respect of disabled peoples limited access to mainstream services), but it had not yet been faced. As a result, then, some aspects of exclusion had been successfully challenged, but others of an equally fundamental nature were not seen to be a relevant part of these initiatives. **It remains an open question whether improved welfare services can be more closely combined with ways of increasing employment.**

These conclusions hold good for the generality of people on whose behalf the changes were made. This leaves the question of specific groups who suffer particular forms of social exclusion. One clear illustration is the situation of immigrants: although they are present in most of the countries studied, sometimes in large numbers, their civil and social rights are not specifically addressed in any of our case studies. In Rostock asylum seekers were burned out of their hostels; the schemes devised catered for groups similar to those who did the burning, but not their victims. Given that immigrants are especially likely to suffer from social exclusion - and, indeed, may not be classed as citizens or be entitled to receive public services - this is an issue which is unlikely to go away. So it is to the general question of equal opportunities for particularly disadvantaged groups that we now turn.

CHAPTER SIX : Equal Opportunities

Increasing consumer involvement in public services is not a substitute for promoting equal rights, treatment and opportunities for the consumers of public welfare services. Consumer involvement initiatives which are concerned to combat the stigma and exclusion facing many citizens need to be developed in a way which reflects a commitment to promoting equal opportunities for all. In building public services which reflect this commitment it is important to bear in mind that the processes which are developed are of fundamental importance. As the European Foundation's previous work has highlighted, in working to reduce inequality generated by social and economic imbalances it is vital to bear in mind that "The ways in which services are provided and delivered are more important than what they are" (EFILWC, 1994).

Equal opportunities commitment in public welfare services must not be confined to issues of service delivery alone. Equal opportunities also need to be delivered in the area of employment practice in public welfare services. The evidence across Europe is that public welfare service organisations are characterised by the fact that whilst women employees predominate in the lowest status positions they are largely missing from the arenas of organisational and political influence. The European Commission's Social Policy White Paper (A Way Forward for the Union) noted that "the objective of equality between women and men will be frustrated if much more rapid progress is not made in the representation of women in public and political bodies" (European Commission, 1994:43).

Any assessment of equal opportunites must pay attention to the impact on women as employees, as well as users, of new initiatives in the public services (EFILWC, op cit, 1994). Women's experiences are therefore one of the major themes of the evidence assembled in the sixteen case studies.

As the European Commission have recently acknowledged in 'A Way Forward for the Union' "Women are not a homogeneous group. Much discrimination comes from the same historical and cultural roots and affects all women. However, policies need also to address differing needs and expectations, for example, disabled, elderly, migrant and/or ethnic minority, young women or those that live in rural areas or inner cities" (1994:41(5)). Such diversity also needs to be considered in relation to the promotion of equal opportunities.

In order to discuss the extent to which the sixteen case studies reflected a commitment to equal opportunities, we audited them for reference to the way in which equal opportunity policies informed their procedures and outcomes in respect to both service delivery and employment practice.

Features of Equal Opportunity

Each case study was examined for evidence of one or more of the following six equal opportunity features:

A   An equal opportunity policy for employment practice

B   An equal opportunity policy for service delivery

C   The incorporation of an equal opportunities dimension in the design of the consumer involvement initiative

D   Equal opportunities targets set by/for front line staff engaged in the initiative

E   Equal opportunities monitoring of the service outcomes of the initiative

F   Equal opportunities monitoring of the employment practice outcomes of the initiative.

A   **Equal opportunity policies in relation to employment practice** were referred to in only two of the agencies associated with the consumer-involvement initiatives. The UK Severnside Benefits Agency had equal opportunity training for staff and an equal opportunities Standing Committee "involving Trade Union Representatives and staff drawn from groups typically likely to experience discrimination - women, people with disabilities, people from ethnic minorities and so on" as part of the formal structure of the organisation. This Agency had also made a commitment to developing an Equal Opportunity Action Plan in relation to both employment practice and service delivery. Italy's Pensione Subito staff were employed by a government agency - INPS - with a Committee for Equal Opportunities which commissioned research into the training and promotion of men and women.

B   **Equal opportunity policies related to service delivery** were rare. The UK Severnside Benefit Agency was developing such a policy. The Amadora Social Security initiative in Portugal reflected a central government social security programme "marked by the principles of greater social justice, better social provision and the promotion of increasing equality of opportunity".

C   **The incorporation of an equal opportunities dimension in the design of the consumer involvement initiative** was rarely in evidence in the case studies. The analysis of both Irish initiatives highlighted that "There has been a lack of awareness in respect of an equal opportunities dimension to consumer-oriented service delivery to date in Ireland." In the QUIP initiative this meant that "No significant attempt was made to incorporate an equal opportunity dimension into the design of the initiative." One outcome of this was that the self-selected members of the QUIP teams greatly under-represented the proportion of women employed at the equivalent levels of the agency.

There were attempts, however, by some projects to make an explicit commitment to redressing inequality for specific groups within the community. For example the Hyldespjaeldet Social Network project had a commitment to promote democracy and equality through community participation in problem solving and within this framework worked with specific disadvantaged groups. The Rostock Arche initiative also focused its work on specific groups including young people in unstable circumstances, lone parents and disabled people. The Wiltshire Community Care Network had an explicit commitment to work with the unequal relationships which exist between service users and professional staff in community care services. This commitment was pursued by developing and supporting the empowerment and involvement of users who were disabled and/or elderly.

However, the fact that the majority of these users and their carers were women was not a dimension which was explicitly addressed in the empowerment work undertaken by this project.

D **Equal opportunities targets set by/for front line staff** were rarely to be found in the initiatives as a means of addressing inequality and disadvantage. Amongst the few that took this approach it is interesting that gender and race were not the focus of the targets set. The Hyldespjaeldet Estate Action project guided by its broad equality commitment targeted groups deemed to be disadvantaged within their community. In this instance the young unemployed, unemployed people with a criminal record, people with mental illness, older people, single parents, children and "drop outs". The Rostock Arche project strove to plan and develop services with the disadvantaged groups they had targeted. The Wiltshire Community Care Users Network made an explicit commitment to addressing the inequality experienced by older and disabled people.

E **Equal opportunity monitoring systems in relation to employment practice** were not well evidenced in the case studies. The exception here was the Severnside Benefits Agency which had "pledged itself to equal opportunities monitoring at all stages of the recruitment process, training and promotion process". Critical to the monitoring of outcome here was the work of an Equal Opportunities Standing Committee.

F **Equal opportunity monitoring systems in relation to service delivery** outcomes were not a key part of project monitoring. In the few initiatives where monitoring the outcome of service delivery was part of the initial project design, an equal opportunities perspective was not apparent. For example in the Beja Health initiative, the monitoring focus was on increasing service to a given population with no consideration of the way in which this might impact on the promotion of equal opportunities amongst service users, or between them and the rest of the population.

Elements of Equal Opportunities in the Case Studies

Research suggests (Beresford and Croft, 1993) that in striving to develop accessible, appropriate, adequate and accountable services, consumer-oriented initiatives must take full account of the following four elements of equal opportunity policy:

* *Equal access* - bringing down barriers and opening up communication.

* *Equal shares* - ensuring that the proportion of consumers (in all service areas) and those employed in the services (at all levels) reflect those in the wider community served.

* *Equal treatment* - striving to develop appropriately diverse service responses to members of minority groups in order to ensure that the disadvantage and discrimination they face are positively addressed.

* *Equal outcomes* - monitoring equality outcomes to inform longer term policy and practice change.

Equal Access

This was understood as being characterised by four dimensions:

Physical access - providing an accessible environment to those with limited mobility, for example, by adapting buildings, integrating and relocating services so that they are locally based, and providing adequate facilities for those with young children;

Language - enabling people to communicate on equal terms;

Psychological access - ensuring that a service is delivered in a manner which is welcoming to those from different backgrounds and cultures;

Time - providing services which are available at times to suit users and give sufficient time to address users' concerns.

TABLE 6.1 Equal access and the case studies	1	2	3	4	5	6	7	8	9	10	11	12	13	14	15	16
Physical		*		*	*	*	*	*	*	*	*	*	*	*	*	*
Language					*								*			*
Psycholog.	*			*		*			*			*	*	*	*	
Time							*		*		*					

Key to case studies

1 Italy, Pensione Subito
2 Greece, IKA Pensions
3 Germany, Prosoz
4 Ireland, QUIP Disability Pensions
5 UK, Severnside Benefits Agency
6 Ireland, Ballyfermot One-Stop Shop
7 Portugal, Amadora Social Security
8 Italy, Tribunale del Malato

9 Portugal, Beja Health
10 Greece, Kapi Old Peoples Centre
11 Denmark, Odense Home Care
12 France, L'Alliance Elderly Centre
13 UK, Wiltshire Community Care
14 France, Nantes Habitat
15 Germany, Rostock Arche
16 Denmark, Hyldespjaeldet

As the Table 6.1 shows, the majority of case studies provided evidence that consumer-oriented initiatives result in an increase in **physical access** to services. Critically for many this was a result of combining service integration with decentralisation of service location. However, this approach did not always have an equal access outcome for all consumers.

For example the Ballyfermot One-Stop Shop project noted that whilst an integrated relocation to a local site had increased access for some consumers, it created barriers to access for others. "The lack of a lift makes the private interview rooms and the Community Welfare Officer located on the second floor inaccessible to wheelchair users. Similarly women, who are the main clients of the Community Welfare Office have to carry young children and buggies or prams to the upstairs waiting area and no public toilet facilities are available in the building".

In the Prosoz initiative, plans for more welcoming waiting rooms with facilities for mothers and young children were abandoned in the face of demands for more office space for staff. In contrast, issues of access for mothers with children in hospital were part of the successful advocacy work undertaken by the Tribunale project.

There was very scant evidence that the issue of increasing **language access** was a focus of concern in the case studies. No reference was made in any case study to the availability of service information in translation for consumers from ethnic minority groups, although in the UK, the Severnside Benefits Agency were reviewing this together with a consideration of the use of interpreters. The case studies which provided evidence that they were addressing this dimension of access focused on communication with consumers who were disabled and those who had limited literacy skills. For example, the Wiltshire Community Care Users Network held meetings "in venues which provided a full range of assistance to participation and communication and were organised with a structured framework and friendly atmosphere that facilitated participation". These approaches included, for example, clear, jargon-free information.

Literacy issues were identified and addressed by the Severnside Benefits Agency which provided assistance for those with reading and writing difficulties and the Hyldespjaeldet Social Network project which identified literacy problems amongst project workers and took steps to provide them with assistance in order to address the inequality they experienced. The Beja health service made a point of simplifying and demythologising language.

In relation to addressing **psychological** barriers to access there were no examples of initiatives which specifically addressed the needs of individuals from communities with diverse cultures. However the two UK initiatives cited in Table 1 provided examples of taking positive steps to provide a more psychologically welcoming environment. In the Severnside Benefit Agency the reception area was designed to create facilities for women with young children. The Wiltshire Community Care User Network gave priority to creating supportive environments in meeting venues which promoted the empowerment of disabled people through help with "overcoming (often considerable) fear, speaking out, being heard, understood and responded to by others in a similar situation".

The approach of the Pensione Subito initiative provided an important example of using the introduction of new technology to provide a more welcoming service style. Staff engaged in identifying an individual's pension rights invited consumers to sit alongside the front line staff while they calculated their entitlement on computer screen displays. The Rostock Arche project's approach to going out and about to meet excluded citizens on their own territory to discuss service developments and possible service use provided another example of attempts to overcome psychological barriers to service access (outreach activities).

Time emerged as a feature in the Amadora Social Security project where the largely female staff group took a decision to change the standard office opening and closing hours in order to take account of their lives as women with domestic responsibilities. A motivating factor in the development of the Odense Integrated Care project was to deliver a 24 hour needs-led service to older disabled people living in the community.

Equal Shares

In relation to employment practice the majority of case studies highlighted the dominance of women as front line service workers. In some initiatives the changes that had been set in motion had increased the number of front line jobs available to women as well as the part such women played in making decisions about service provision (eg Beja Health and Amadora Social Security; Odense Integrated Care). However, few projects ventured beyond the front line and looked in any detail at the impact of these changes on the share that women employees took in decision-making at higher levels of public services and within the political domain. Given the importance of such decision making forums in promoting the kind of "top down" change which shaped many of the initiatives in this study this omission raised a number of important questions about equal shares. Several of the national reports (eg Germany, Ireland, Italy, Portugal and the UK) noted a marked absence of women at the higher levels of decision-making. There appeared to be little response made in the sixteen case studies to this state of affairs. An exception here was the Prosoz initiative where a women's training group was established at the request of project staff. This step was taken because training was identified in this initiative as an important way to address the under-representation of women in public service management.

The case studies provided virtually no evidence relating to other issues of equal shares in employment practice. Only the Severnside Benefits Agency initiative drew attention to the relative lack of staff recruited from local black or ethnic minority communities. No evidence was available from any project about the representation of people with disabilities amongst those in paid employment. However, where projects succeeded in drawing consumers into active service provision, planning and training in a paid and/or unpaid capacity, (eg Hyldespjaeldet Social Network, Rostock Arche and Wiltshire Community Care Users Network) then a visibly more representative group of workers was established as the direct result of the initiative.

As for equal shares in relation to service provision, the dominance of women as service users was noted in several of the projects. These women were seeking resources to meet their own needs and/or those of members of their households. However it was not always the case that the profile of service use reflected "equal shares". In the Kapi project, for example, it was noted that despite the dominance of women in the target population of older people, more men than women in fact accessed the service. In contrast it was noted that the Rostock Arche project became a 'catalyst' for the development of services provided "by women for women" which was planned to reach groups outside the project's original remit. The Tribunale initiative found itself undertaking a significant amount of advocacy work on behalf of women who were mothers of young children receiving health care as well as women who were carers.

References to women's use of services tended in all studies to be references to a homogeneous group of potential or actual service users. The diversity amongst women related to, for example, age, disability, race and religion, was largely unacknowledged in the case study evaluations. This outcome may in part reflect the way in which researchers focused on women as a disadvantaged group as well as the lack of relevant information from the case studies. However it may also be the case that such a perspective reflects

91

the way in which the service providing agencies identify women's issues without paying attention to diversity amongst women users - who are in fact drawn from, and are mediating on behalf of, a diversity of disadvantaged groups and communities.

Both of the Danish projects as well as the German Rostock Arche provided some important insights into the problems experienced by community-based initiatives committed to simultaneously extending equal shares to a range of excluded groups. For example, in the Hyldespjaeldet Social Network a group of residents who were former psychiatric patients were initially targeted as potential service users. But at an early stage of the project this group became identified as potentially damaging to both the image of the community served by the project and to the project itself. As a result this group was excluded from the mainstream of the project's activity and their needs were identified as requiring separate, specialist and segregated service response.

Equal Treatment

A systematic consideration of this area was hampered by the fact that most of the initiatives failed to engage explicitly with the issue of diversity amongst consumer groups and service responses to diversity. The emphasis in all of the case studies tended to be on general service improvements which were often assumed to be the way to deliver equal treatment for all. For example, in the Portuguese Amadora Social Security project staff explicitly stated that they avoided treating groups of consumers differently. "On the question of priority treatment for the disabled, pregnant women and the elderly, it was stated that these groups were given preferential treatment only in exceptional circumstances. The pleasant and comfortable physical environment at the office meant there was no justification for offering preferential treatment". Such responses were not based on any researched consideration of whether it is possible for a "same" treatment approach to deliver equality of treatment to very diverse groups of service users.

Equal Outcomes

The majority of initiatives had not been designed to incorporate monitoring and evaluation as an ongoing process. For most projects the evaluation conducted for the Foundation provided the only evidence with which to begin to review outcomes. Where projects had been evaluated systematically, for example Beja Health in Portugal and Prosoz in Bremen, the outcome measures did not extend to a consideration of equal opportunities. The emphasis was on such factors as increasing service coverage, turnover, technical efficiency and targeting. The concerns appeared to be service and resource driven. So, for example, in relation to the Odense Integrated Care Scheme it was noted that "equalising of the use of resources between the institutions and people's own homes... resulted in fewer resources being available for the sheltered houses and nursing home, since the staff began to provide help to people in their own homes in the institution's neighbourhood." Whether such an outcome could be considered as improving equality of opportunity or treatment in relation to service users was not addressed.

Summary and Conclusions

The experiences gathered across these case studies provide a rich source from which to identify the directions in which public welfare services need to develop their equal opportunity agendas. Many of the initiatives in this study succeeded in delivering a measure of improved access and responsiveness to service users and as a result some members of disadvantaged and excluded groups found themselves in receipt of a service which they might have otherwise been denied.

However, this equal opportunity audit of the case study material suggests that most of these sixteen service initiatives were developed in public service organisations in which there was no major commitment to equal opportunities issues. As a result the outcomes they delivered failed to engage clearly with the inequalities experienced by members of diversely disadvantaged communities. No initiative worked to combine a commitment to equal opportunities policy at agency level with targets established by front line staff, shared and developed in partnership with consumers. Some projects had elements of a limited "top down" commitment to equal opportunities. Some provided evidence of a limited "bottom up" commitment to addressing equal opportunity issues for some groups of consumers and/or staff. There was no evidence of sustained monitoring in this area and subsequent equal opportunity policy and practice development directed at working towards establishing equality indicators for services and increasing equality outcomes.

Consumer-oriented initiatives have a potentially important role to play in working towards a more equal Europe. This study suggests that if this is to be realised there is a critical need to identify, select for study, as well as design, user-oriented initiatives which reflect a sustained commitment to equal opportunities, treatment and outcome for the users of public sector services. This commitment needs to extend and strengthen its focus on women by acknowledging and responding to diversity amongst users and employees in respect to race, religion, age and disability. Such a commitment to promoting equality is the key to ensuring that public welfare services strengthen their user-responsiveness and in doing so find ways of positively contributing to "increasing economic and social cohesion and fighting against the exclusion of disadvantaged groups" (EFILWC, 1994).

CHAPTER SEVEN :   The Process of Change

This chapter changes the focus: instead of analysing outcomes, it contains a commentary on the process of change itself, so as to draw lessons for planning future initiatives. It begins with a discussion of the factors which precipitated changes and facilitated their successful enactment; it goes on to examine whether the impetus came from the top, bottom or outside the organisations concerned and what implications this had; the type of change is then explored; finally it discusses the roles played by staff and their unions, and then by consumers in making things happen.

Catalysts and Facilitators

All of the **general pressures for change** identified earlier (Chapter 1) can be seen at work in our case studies. A common sequence has featured a phase of expansion as the 'push' factors of rising expectations and socio-demographic change (especially ageing), leading to a growing recognition of diversity, have combined with the 'pull' factors of technical progress. Economic retrenchment has then brought a growing pressure for cost containment at the same time as an increased demand for social protection services. One element of this, the threat to social order and cohesion, acted as a background factor in a number of cases, but came to the forefront in Rostock and Hyldespjaeldet. This new stimulus has, however, overlain rather than replaced the pressures for growth. Increased efficiency, new technology and managerial reforms have then followed as a first attempt to resolve the dilemmas, combined with a more or less stringent attempt to transfer responsibility for some forms of social protection back to the individual or family. It is at around this stage of development that most of our case studies began. Many commentators have, of course, argued that we have now reached a stage of more radical re-invention of government, as the pressures noted above become more intense and the solutions implemented to date prove insufficient.

So much for the general picture. We have noted however that the types of welfare state in which our case studies took place, as well as their stage of development, differ widely, even if there are some common elements in their current trajectories. The timing at which new stages have impinged has also varied. The problems are perhaps greater in those emergent welfare states in which the infrastructure was not fully established before retrenchment began to bite: and they are shown to extreme in the new federal states of Germany. While this situation is atypical within our sample, it is probably the best representation of the widespread challenges within Eastern and Central Europe, so that any lessons here warrant particular attention.

The shadow which **trends** cast into the future can act as an important catalyst. Often, too, senses of both **opportunity** and **crisis** seem to combine to create the conditions for change - the crises in our cases being the rejection of old models among professionals (Beja Health, Wiltshire community care), the threat of greater professional and managerial power (Wiltshire again, and the Italian Tribunals) or the multiple crises and opportunities of re-unification (Rostock).

Another major impetus concerns new **visions and identities.** Just as the residents of Hyldespjaeldet believed in themselves, so the new self-identities nurtured in the wider disability movement (which had re-defined disability not as something inherent within individuals, but as the consequence of disabling social arrangements) strongly influenced the motivation and behaviour of key actors in Wiltshire. Initial success in establishing networks could then both feed on itself and legitimate the partnership with staff whose views were similarly converted. Of course, the visions are not only broadly based, but can be significantly enhanced by compatible detailed policy models imported from elsewhere. In Beja the model came from the World Health Organisation. In Rostock it came immediately from the twin town of Bremen, having begun elsewhere. In both instances people who acted as **policy evangelists and entrepreneurs** were vital to its successful adoption. This happened to be a leading insider in Beja, but an outside consultant, with inside support, filled the role in Rostock. It is crucial, however, that they have the support of powerful **sponsors**, if they lack that power themselves. That might be the senior management of the agency, as in Pensione Subito, Prosoz and Severnside, or key politicians (Rostock, both French cases and New Ionia, Greece). In either case, change of leaders or their pre-occupation with other matters can have adverse consequences (Greek Kapis and QUIP, Ireland).

The Locus and Direction of Change

The vast majority of the initiatives concerned formal government agencies (see Table 7.1), although the Italian Patients' Rights Tribunals and the Hyldespjaeldet project emanated from outside government - one to exert influence upon it and the other in lieu of government action. In other instances, such as Rostock and Wiltshire, non-governmental agencies were involved as partners. The level of governance is inevitably a reflection of the distribution of functions in the various countries, the norm being that pensions and social security are handled centrally, whereas responsibility for services in kind is devolved. This allows greater scope for experimentation but can place limits on the widespread adoption of successful change. Equally government rules and actions can either facilitate local change (Rostock) or hinder it (Beja health).

Irrespective of these varying levels of governance, the majority of changes were initiated from the top downwards. Sometimes this would be in conjunction with actors nearer the periphery, either in partnership or sequentially, with the centre promulgating the initial ideas and the periphery taking them up and making them happen. Specific grants and incentive funds, to be discussed later, are important facilitators.

Top down changes are frequently based on managerial initiatives occasioned by a crisis of excess demand over possible supply under current production methods and fiscal ceilings. New technologies of management and service delivery are seen as the means of escape from this dilemma. Top down changes inevitably involve the development and imposition of common patterns. Thus the political and managerial leaders have a role not only in resourcing the initiative, but also in championing it and managing the change process. Frequently, however, the enthusiastic involvement of staff at lower levels is vital to making things happen. Here, the tactics may be to create a cascade of change, leaving decisions as to its detailed form to those nearer to the action.

TABLE 7.1 What sort of change and from where does it emanate?

	Cash services											Services in kind				
	Pensione Subito	IKA Pensions	Prosoz	QUIP	Severnside	Ballyfermot	Amadora	Tribunale	Beja Health	Kapi	Odense	L'Alliance	Wiltshire	Nantes Habitat	Rostock Arche	Hyldesp jaeldet
Governance																
National	**	**		**	**	**	**			*				*		
Regional/local			**						**	*	**	*	*	*		
Non-governmental								**				*	*			**
Locus and Direction																
Top down	**	**	**	*	**	**	*		*	**	**	**		**		
Mixed/Partnership				*			*		*				*		*	
Grass roots								**					*		*	**
Dominant type of change																
Reform	*	*	*	*	*	*	*	***	*	*	*	*		*		
Innovation	*	*	*	*	*	*	*	***	**	*	*	*	**	*	**	**

The role of staff will be discussed later, but it is important to note here that the failure to sustain support for changes once championed can lead to cynicism and disillusion - as was the case to some degree in the Irish pensions Quality Improvement Programme, the Greek pensions reform and is threatened for the Greek old peoples centres. Conversely the backing of new ventures, especially at crisis points, can provide the space and security for even high risk changes to succeed. That backing may be in the form of political as well as financial support (eg Rostock Arche).

Some programmes involve a **partnership** between those in formal leadership positions and other staff or outsiders. Patterns vary considerably: a formal initiative recruits junior partners (QUIP); a person in a leadership role uses his charisma to persuade staff to join him and shakes free enough outside resources to achieve 'a break with the established order at all levels' (Beja).

Where voluntary organisations and grassroots groups join with public bodies to develop a programme of action (as in Rostock), the management of influence is a key to making things happen. This may entail a willingness by public officials to take on new roles and new ways of behaving. The emphasis seems to be upon individuals or small-scale 'policy communities' seizing opportunities, shaking free resources and developing loose implementation networks to construct programmes. Inevitably the risks of failure are greater and mutual trust in the competence and goodwill of partners to achieve a shared vision is a critical ingredient. The opportunities open to users as partners and the responsibilities upon them are proportionately greater: and frequently the funding basis has to be adapted imaginatively to provide the security and infrastructure support needed. Here, too, there is an opportunity for closer alliances between users and higher level government bodies in influencing change.

It is much rarer among our case studies to find a fully **bottom-up** approach, in which new schemes are generated from the grass roots - the relative disadvantage of the major users and the lack of institutional support and resources being obvious reasons. Those that come closest reflect the diversity likely to arise: the Hyldespjaeldet Social Network project is limited to a local community; the Italian patients' tribunals have grown into a national social movement, but are locally variable in the level, style, content and influence of their activities. In such instances new visions of the possible are vital. Hyldespjaeldet's residents were convinced that they themselves could make a difference. The Patients' Rights Tribunal owed much to dissatisfaction within services, but also to the flowering of popular belief in holistic medicine and the perceived need to reclaim health from professionals, which was allied with an existing movement to reclaim democracy from politicians. In this way a unifying call could receive the support of an established institution.

Types of Change

Virtually all change involves a mix of gradual development of existing practices, doing similar sorts of things in different ways (reform) and doing new things (innovation). Table 7.1 seeks to depict the balance between reform and innovation; the challenge of change differs in each case. For simple development, resources are the dominant constraining factor. **Reform** initiatives face greater challenges concerning their technical and administrative feasibility and must also overcome the dynamic conservatism which organisations and the people in them need to exhibit in the struggle to maintain a steady state - hence the balancing of competing objectives, extensive consultation and coalition-building, while testing out feasibility. Judgements as to the scope of the change and its relationship to other developments can be important to its success: the Italian pensions reform was initially limited to the payments sections, leaving those concerned with entitlements until later; local demonstration projects were chosen in the Irish and British social security reforms. It was not always possible to accommodate all interests, however: the shift to natural remedies in Beja, Portugal, raised the continued opposition of the pharmaceutical companies.

Innovations may encounter less resistance because there are fewer vested interests. However, they may go beyond the existing legitimacy and competence of the organisation as well as facing major challenges as to their feasibility (eg Rostock Arche). Frequently, then, people have to take risks, although they may be contained and localised.

Staff and Trades Unions as Key Actors

The importance of the high level of involvement by staff and their representatives in many cases, and the heavy demands placed upon their creativity, skill, enthusiasm and resilience has already been detailed. What, however, was the nature of their involvement? Did they promote the change or respond to initiatives from above or outside? How heavily involved were they in its design? To what extent did it depend upon them taking responsibility for its implementation or changing their working practices? Table 7.2 suggests that their initial involvement depends on the origin and direction of the change, but that they are normally crucial to its successful implementation.

Within **top-down changes** the staff contribution tends not to be in the conception or broad design of initiatives, but in their detailed development and/or introduction: they have to make the changes work. Top-down planning makes it possible to design jobs, procedures, incentive systems and consultation mechanisms which reinforce the desired changes. Indeed most of the top-down initiatives either recruited staff representatives as junior partners in detailed design, or consulted them extensively. The work of trades unions, acting on behalf of those whose jobs were to be substantially changed, as well as those whose work disappeared, proved to be vital in several instances (such as Pensione Subito and Prosoz). That work was in several directions: ensuring that staff interests were properly considered in the detailed design of changes; reassuring a sometimes suspicious workforce that it was safe to become involved; assisting in training; and calling for proper evaluation (as in Odense).

Clearly, **adequate training** to use new technology and to provide a more open and responsive service to consumers is critical. A personalised service for example, also means potentially more exposure to dissatisfaction. This is especially the case where the bringer of bad news is seen also to have greater discretion over the decision. Such a risk is reduced by long traditions of deference towards public services, or low expectations of them. However, consumer-oriented initiatives attack those attitudes and also the de-personalisation and anonymity which accompanies them.

101

TABLE 7.2 Staff as key actors

	Cash services										Services in kind					
	Pensione Subito	IKA Pensions	Prosoz	QUIP	Severnside	Ballyfermot	Amadora	Tribunal	Beja Health	Kapi	Odense	L'Alliance	Wiltshire	Nantes Habitat	Rostock Arche	Hyldespjaeldet
Entrepreneurs of change									*	*					*	
Partners in design				*	*		*		*	*		*	*		*	
Consulted over design			*			*			*	*				*		
Delegated responsibilities for implementation	*	*	*	*	*	*			*	*	*	*		*		
Job enlargement and change	*	*	*	*	*	*	*		*		*	*	*	*		
Special role of women							*					*				
Reacting to external initiatives								*				*	*		*	

102

The employment of local staff in decentralised integrated offices, and the expansion of their work at the front line, adds to potential pressures. In several instances, then, staff reported both strongly favourable views on the improvements in service and in their own working conditions, and also growing anxiety about heavy workloads, the exercise of discretion (especially where there was an element of rationing) and the pressures arising from being close to the customer (too close for comfort sometimes), both inside and outside the office. These issues came to the fore in the Severnside (UK) and Ballyfermot (Ireland) cases. However, the Italian pensions workers were also under pressure to resolve consumers' difficulties with other, less accessible sections of their agency: consumers do not see their problems in the neat organisational patterns of bureaucracies. Hence, the need to say 'no', not just nicely, but quickly and safely, and to assist in the re-direction of problems, is likely to increase. The Amadora office, combining not only pension and social security services, but also services in kind, including charitable equipment, therefore provided not only a better overall service, but also a less stressful environment for staff.

Of course, the issue is not only to deal with consumers' responses to increased discretion, but also to develop clear guidelines and skills in how to exercise it. One consumer-oriented response to this - the imposition and publication of rules - does not fit easily into the mix of objectives which provoke many of the changes, and it is likely to be resisted (eg Prosoz). Without clear guidance - and means of public challenge - overburdened staff are likely to develop ad hoc, privatised rules of thumb to defend themselves against the pain of such discretion.

Overall, then, the staff contribution to top-down change and its continued implementation should not be underestimated. They have to keep the service going during the changes; they have to make the changes; jobs at the frontline have been enlarged and conflicting pressures to ration services and to be close to the consumer have been incorporated; and the success of the changes is judged by the quality at the frontline.

The harnessing and nurturing of skills, enthusiasm and more productive working practices has been a major means of overcoming resource constraint. Here the previously underutilised abilities of workers in front-line positions - including their flexibility as 'patchworkers' - stitching together workable solutions in uncertain situations and accepting less than secure working conditions in doing so - have provided the chief ingredients. These skills have also been at a premium in other examples of top-down change, where staff are left to develop their own solutions to multi-professional and multi-agency co-ordination, in the absence of management attention to the problem. As in the Greek Kapi case, external threats to resources can quickly threaten joint working by encouraging defensiveness.

In those circumstances where **the dynamic for change is mixed** and people from lower levels of the agency, or outside it, are incorporated as significant actors, the pressure on staff can be of a different order. The case studies reveal two types of situation. First, non-conformists in the organisation promote changes which run counter to established ways of doing things (eg Beja health). They believe that these will provide more effective services for the public, even if they cut across the interests of the organisation or powerful groups within it.

The second situation is when desired changes are beyond the scope of a public agency and political, administrative and technical leaders join forces in informal coalitions to garner sufficient resources and support. Here the initiative tends to operate outside, rather than in spite of, standard operating procedures.

Nevertheless, the functions to be filled are similar. Frequently, staff are to be found in the roles of evangelists preaching reform and innovation, of policy entrepreneurs stitching together coalitions and funding, of development engineers taking risks and taking on extra work in order to make the vision real. In these circumstances, jobs, procedures and even rules may be bent to make spaces for change. The distinctions between staff, users and governors may be blurred. And key people may occupy unorthodox and insecure niches - as researchers, evaluators or paid trainees in order to carry out the necessary work (Rostock Arche). This minimum necessary infrastructure is frequently financed by incentive funding and the lack of fit between its rules and the work seen to be needed on the ground accounts for the unorthodoxy.

If the pressures on staff taking on these roles - and sometimes doing their normal work alongside them - are not to lead to high rates of attrition, support mechanisms, such as high levels of mutual trust, a shared mission, expert advice and influential sponsorship at times of crisis have been shown to be vital.

Where changes occurred from the **bottom up**, outside government agencies, it was far more open and variable. Government agencies and the staff representing them might largely ignore the initiative unless and until it became successful or assumed importance - as in Hyldespjaeldet. Alternatively, staff might ignore, resist, collaborate with or become enthusiastic members of the initiative - as all happened with the Italian Tribunals. In such circumstances, the situation is again likely to be fluid. If the initiative is successful and it gains insider status, there is a process of more or less enthusiastic accommodation to its activities.

Consumers as Key Actors

Popular pressures have frequently created an impetus for change and consumers are at the heart of the whole process. Paradoxically, they are frequently cast as objects of, rather than active participants in, the change process: improvements are planned for them, rather than with them. This is especially the case in **top-down changes.** Here, there were only limited examples of specific surveys either to inform planned change or to evaluate its impacts, while more extensive involvement was even less frequent. Three examples offer contrasting insights. In Bremen the conditions of crucial incentive funding stipulated that consumers be represented and a well organised welfare rights movement was therefore able to claim its place on the planning committee. Nonetheless, they were unable to keep some of their most important claims - such as transparency of assessment criteria - on the reform agenda. In the Severnside benefits office (UK) an attempt to form a consultative consumer forum fell flat initially and was then colonised by formal voluntary sector interests, rather than by the consumers themselves. This mirrors the lessons of more limited consultation exercises: consumers must first have expectations of rights to decent services, and to have explored ideas as to what might be desirable, as a pre-condition for dialogue. And if that dialogue is to be extensive, they need the resources and energy to engage in it, as well as the hope that it might be worthwhile. The mutual support provided by groups of disadvantaged consumers is also amply demonstrated, reinforcing the findings of earlier Foundation studies (EFILWC, 1993). Our third example is more hopeful: in the Greek Kapis a top-down change which incorporated participation and voice within its desired outcomes was more successful than anticipated. Here, of course, extended contact and the possibility of co-production of services in kind were facilitative.

These examples suggest that some more extended mechanisms of consumer consultation and involvement at the point of use are more appropriate to services in kind, than cash services, but also point to the importance of power relations. A further question is the extent to which the consumerist outcomes detailed earlier will themselves create the conditions within which further involvement can later take place: we must remember that the case studies are snapshots or brief historical accounts of dynamic events.

Some of the studies in which the impetus for change came from **mixed directions** replicate the experience of top-down changes. The partnerships or sequences of events involved politicians and staff, with any consumer involvement being as a consequence of initiatives rather than an integral and original part of them.

It seems from the evidence here that users need to possess the resources thought necessary for overall success, or powers to disrupt, before they are engaged as partners. It is worth reiterating here that power can be allocated to them in the form of grant aid conditions from higher levels of government (Prosoz, Bremen and Rostock Arche). In most instances of partnership the link is to particular interest communities, such as single parents or disabled people. However, there are subtle variations between groups: in Rostock the young unemployed and able-bodied people, especially men, were more likely than disabled or elderly people to be given roles similar to those of paid staff.

Involvement, then, may be important to users, not only in the chance to shape services to their needs and desires, but also to give them access to paid employment, since the roles of user and provider can be blurred. Equally, it places heavy demands upon them, which are balanced by somewhat limited infrastructural supports (Wiltshire Community Care). If they are incorporated into paid positions, they are especially vulnerable to short-term funding and also the risk of having to do work which does not fit their formal job descriptions (Rostock Arche). In these circumstances both the sponsorship of powerful individuals and the availability of supportive expertise and advice seem to have been important conditions for the success of partnerships. It should be pointed out that these indications are based upon a limited number of successful initiatives (although other experience supports them). We have no examples of substantial failure from which to learn, although there were instances of high levels of attrition among some individuals involved (e.g. Rostock). The more that partnerships are with vulnerable people, living hazardous lives in inauspicious circumstances, the more important those infrastructural supports become.

Membership is cast more widely in the two clearest instances of control and self-management - the community action in Hyldespjaeldet and Italian Patients' Tribunals: they provide the closest link between people as consumers of individual services and people as citizens with wider concerns for the quality of life for others, as well as themselves. Having the strongest action element, the Danish example raises most questions about the 'ownership' of changes by public authorities. Is community self-help an example of partnership or of abandonment and abdication - just as, on an individual level, people may increasingly be expected to manage social care within their own personal networks? It also raises questions about the representativeness of indigenous social action and the mechanisms by which people give an account of and are held to account for their actions. Many of the rules of the game are unclear: this extends to rules about being good employers of staff recruited by self-help initiatives.

Such problems are less in evidence when empowerment takes the form of a powerful voice, exercised upon established public services. The Italian Patients' Tribunals represent empowerment as citizens through the political and legal processes, but eschewing the political parties. The main link to traditional representative democracy arises where politicians see the changes as responding to the needs of their voting constituents (Nantes, Greek Kapis). Otherwise the exercise of citizen influence is not well established in the case examples. The Italian case, then, represents an extreme example of a broader phenomenon - the rise and powerfulness of new social movements based upon the consumption of important public services, as well as the problems which traditional forms of representative democracy face in adapting to them. Nonetheless, such initiatives offer the best opportunity of exercising collective influence, so that when people consume services as individuals, they do so under conditions of their own choosing.

National Policy Impacts

Finally, we complete the picture by linking back briefly to the changes at national level described in Chapter 2, using for this purpose the types of change set out in Chapter 3 (**Access, Choice, Voice** and **Accountability**).

Access is mainly a focus for action at local level; but **choice** and ways of extending it has been an objective of policy at national level in several of the countries in which studies have been undertaken. At the same time, the nature of most of the 'mature' welfare systems is such as to greatly limit the scope for choice between service providers, or even within public welfare sector provision. This is a weakness in current programmes which will need to be addressed, for two reasons. First, both the rhetoric and practice of the 'new public management', with its references to the desirability of adopting prevailing practices from the market and enhancing the status of the "customers" of public services elevates choice as a desirable objective for policy. Pressure to do so is reinforced by the perception that choice will also help to enhance efficiency through encouraging competition, either directly or through 'benchmarking' the performance of other agencies. Second, the pressures from consumer organisations and individual users of services are going to push organisations in the direction of providing more choices.

In some instances, individuals are going to want to make their own choices about how they invest their time and energies in caring tasks rather than accept the subordinate roles in the provision of welfare to which the public services have often assigned them in the past. Services which encourage independence rather than reinforcing dependency also enhance choice.

Voice is one means by which consumers can assert their desire to shape their own role in the delivery of welfare. For both staff and consumers, there are a variety of stages in the introduction and development of new programmes at which voices can be raised; and the evidence of the studies indicates that some advantage is already being taken of these opportunities. Networking and alliances involving exchange of experience can increase the impact of the consumer voice; this is particularly important to encourage, because the contributions of consumers often tends to be very specific, either to their own personal situation or to the individual service of which they are users.

However, a gap here is the shortage of systematic coalitions of interests operating at national and European level which would amplify the individual or group voice currently being heard only within specific services or local welfare systems. The existence of state agencies with a particular responsibility for addressing the problems faced by disadvantaged groups may help here; these 'national equality agencies', of which examples exist in several European countries, especially in the UK and Ireland, can make a substantial contribution especially if they act in tandem with groups directly representing the people concerned. However, to be fully effective, such groupings need to be independent of government and seen to be so. It is encouraging that a number of such networks (European Anti-Poverty Network, for example) have emerged over the past few years and begun to play a part in the policy dialogue at European level. The increasingly active involvement of trades unions at this level ensures that the collective voice of the staff affected by (and involved in) new public service initiatives will be heard. Employers are another group whose involvement is likely to be of increasing significance, separately or together with the unions, as 'social partners'. Another potentially important network is professional groups; but although some links exist here too (for example, between social workers) they have not been systematically deployed in debates about the future of social welfare programmes.

The different ways in which voices can be raised so as to exert influence on policy making at all levels also merits further attention. The use of opinion polls and focus groups by public authorities to measure public satisfaction with services is now quite frequent. However, these devices normally structure responses in such a way as to exclude debate on the objectives of policy. If consumer interests are to be fully represented, consideration needs to be given to alternative ways of expressing views. The use of the media (press, radio and television) by citizen groups to promote their own policy proposals is becoming an increasingly common tactic. Pressure groups often commission their own opinion polls.

Accountability is the fourth major dimension. This is a complex concept which takes many different forms. Accountability by those providing services to those who are receiving it (the consumers) may cut across the responsibility of managers to the funding agency and ultimately to the citizens whose taxes provide the funds. Reforms in the public sector in some European countries have created new structures that stand some way apart from traditional government departments; in others, semi-autonomous agencies have always had the main responsibility for service delivery. These agencies are not accountable in the traditional democratic sense. Voluntary associations and the private sector are now taking on an increased role. In these circumstances, contracts may provide a measure of accountability by service providers from outside the state sector but it is one which does not always adequately reflect the interests of the consumers. Setting standards for service delivery and the creation of mechanisms through which performance is assessed and quality maintained can make an important contribution here.

Different traditions of public service assign different roles to elected officials; their close involvement in decisions about resource allocation can be either an asset - reflecting democratic lines of accountability - or a source of problems, leading to politically or personally biased decisions, clientelism or even corruption, depending on the context. Democratic accountability can also be exercised in other forms; the participatory democracy of the neighbourhood rather than the representative democracy of the ballot box. In sum, the need is to distinguish different forms and determine which is most appropriate for the circumstances and best reflects the interests of the different groups and individuals with legitimate interests in the outcome.

Summary and Conclusions

We have seen, from the evidence of the case studies, that the factors precipitating change - mostly those identified in Chapter 1 (social and demographic change, rising expectations, technological progress, cost containment and increased demand) - have both precipitated crises and produced opportunities. A variety of new visions and initiatives have been brought to bear; but mostly the direction of change has been top-down, based upon managerial initiatives but often involving partnerships.

The types of change vary - reforms of existing programmes or innovations; and staff and trades unions have often been key in the process. Issues of the provision of adequate training and harnessing skills and enthusiasm in the cause of achieving constructive change have frequently arisen. Consumers have also featured either as individual actors, or as participants in new social movements.

At national levels, some of the changes taking place are promoting progress in the discussion of the four main aspects of consumer involvement identified in the model for change. Key lessons that stand out include the importance of developing networks for implementation at national and European level and the reinforcement of democratic accountability.

CHAPTER EIGHT :   Conclusions

Context

At the beginning of this report, a number of the most important social problems now facing the European Union were identified as well as some basic principles that should inform the way in which these problems might now be addressed. These 'project key themes' emphasised that:

*   social exclusion persists and affects people in all EU countries regardless of the stage of development of those countries or their type of public welfare system;

*   any reform of public welfare services highlights a wide variety of issues that affect a range of groups with legitimate separate interests in the outcome through their involvement in the delivery or receipt of services (consumers, staff, providers, policy makers and citizens);

*   no systematic attention has been paid in public welfare service reform to equal opportunities policies in their widest sense, and in particular little attention has been paid to gender issues, despite the significant role of women in service provision and in the management of poverty in the home and local community.

In addition to confirming the central relevance of these themes, evidence from the Foundation's research has shown that:

*   new programmes to improve service quality and consumer responsiveness have consistently suffered from problems of lack of continuity, underfunding and even withdrawal of resources; and

*   insufficient attention has been paid to issues of monitoring and evaluation and use of their results, with significant consequences for the extension, transfer and dissemination of good and successful practice.

113

Action

To address these issues successfully will involve taking action at a number of different levels:

- European Union;
- Member States;
- regions, cities and neighbourhoods

and will require the involvement of a variety of actors:

- European Union institutions and organisations;
- national governments;
- regional and local governments;
- politicians at all levels;
- employers and trade unions;
- NGOs and voluntary associations;
- community groups;
- informal networks, families and individual citizens.

The various roles of these actors will be strongly influenced by the differences in local, national and international competencies in the area of public welfare services.

Challenges

The Foundation's research, in particular the case studies, has shown it is feasible and practicable to improve quality and accessibility of public welfare services, eliminate excessive delays, increase dialogue with users and staff, and improve the quality of working conditions and work environment. However this account of recent experience at national and local level has also shown that further initiatives at any of the different levels by the various actors, will need to address a number of important challenges. There are still many deficiencies in public welfare services, such as bureaucratic and monolithic structures, complex and opaque procedures, poor quality management, untrained staff, and a lack of democratic control and accountability. Further improvements to increase the quality and responsiveness of these services, and to develop their contribution to tackling problems of social exclusion, will require greater recognition of the following:-

1. The impact of modernisation and of current social, economic and demographic trends, in particular increased pressures on traditional structures of social support and caring;

2. Demoralisation, apathy and alienation of disadvantaged individuals and local communities, resulting from prolonged experience of social and economic exclusion and of remote, impersonal and inefficient service bureaucracies;

3. A frequent absence of full citizens' rights and appropriate systems of democratic accountability;

4. A general lack of user participation in public service policy formulation and implementation, and the specific difficulties faced in this regard by those most dependent on these services - disadvantaged and excluded individuals and families;

5. Inadequate recognition and undervaluing of the contribution of front line staff (frequently women) and the lack of involvement of staff and/or their unions in the development, implementation and monitoring of change programmes and initiatives;

6. The need for sufficient resources and reliability of support for improvement in public services. Even when central policies are adopted at the highest levels, sufficient attention to implementation and continuity may be lacking;

Finally, while issues of economy, efficiency and effectiveness are as important in public services as they are in the private sector, public services must also be concerned with issues of equity, accountability and democratic control. In private services increased demand will generally lead to increased supply, but for public services, an increase in demand, such as that which has been very apparent in the whole welfare area, leads to calls for prioritisation and rationing. The whole question of the allocation of scarce public resources to competing groups is in essence what democratic politics are about. The tasks facing providers in public services are thus complex and problematic and require greater transparency and extended dialogue.

Recommendations and Guidelines for Future Action

This report pointed earlier to the wide diversity of systems and practices in the various public welfare structures across the European Union, in particular the differing roles of national, regional and local governments, the private and voluntary sectors in service planning, management and delivery. These recommendations and guidelines are therefore likely to have different implications for the various levels and actors, according to national traditions and procedures. However on the basis of the evidence gathered in the course of the Foundation's research, the following are suggested as key issues which require attention in future developments in public welfare services if they are to lead to more responsive and consumer-friendly models of action, and contribute to the building of economic and social cohesion.

The Role of Consumers/Users

1. There should be a greater recognition of **consumers as active partners** with service providers and a systematic adoption of a consumer perspective in future reforms and innovations.

2. Given the alienation and apathy referred to earlier, efforts should be made to **create stronger consumer awareness** and perceptions of the right to access good quality services provided in an equitable and accountable way and to be involved in the process of developing such services. This is particularly important in countries where the consumer movement and traditions of self-help and voluntary activity are weakly developed.

3. There may be little collective capacity for organisation amongst users, especially those from the most vulnerable and disadvantaged groups in society, who are highly dependent on public welfare services. In this case it will be especially important to **develop the pre-conditions for user involvement and empowerment**. Only when users see themselves as having a right to expect quality services and have the ability to make demands and expect responses will they develop the confidence and collective identity around which they can organise as citizens as well as consumers. Support could include funding and training for user organisations; appointment of user network development officers; developing the capacity for the system to facilitate user involvement at all levels, and providing an organisational culture that welcomes criticism and contributions from users.

4. **Surveys of user satisfaction** can be an important part of on-going monitoring and evaluation of welfare services and can help to identify areas requiring improvement. However, they are not a substitute for user participation.

5. More assistance may be required for users who are permanently or temporarily unable to speak for themselves. In this case support should be given to the development of **advocacy services** and the use of other intermediaries particularly in the voluntary and non-governmental sectors. There is a need here to distinguish between such intermediaries who are service deliverers, possibly under contract to public authorities, and those whose main function is to represent users and exert pressure for change.

6. Availability of non-technical, clear and comprehensible **information** provides a crucial basis for consumer access, choice and consultation.

7. **Alliances** with other key actors, especially staff, can help to promote and implement improvements, but there is also need for recognition that the interests of the different actors may not be identical or compatible, which points to the necessity for dialogue, consultation and negotiation.

8. More room and support (financial and non-material) should be made available for **self-help and local community based initiatives** which have been shown to successfully supplement public services particularly in providing more sensitive, tailored approaches to deal with the complex and multidimensional nature of the problems facing the most disadvantaged and excluded in our society. Greater delegation of delivery and control has important implications for role changes for public authorities and for the need to ensure equity and accountability.

9. The **press and media** can play a role in the development of a culture of user protest and engagement with public authorities. This may be significant where there is a general tendency among users to be passive or defensive, faced with a tradition of immutable public service structures and great inequalities of power between users and public service providers. The media could also play a bigger role in information campaigns aimed at public service users.

10. The lack of user participation and consultation particularly affects **women and ethnic minorities** who tend to have much less influence on, and access to, decision making.

11. There is a need for greater understanding of the relationship between **consumerism and citizenship**. The denial of legitimate access to public services equates to a denial of access to full citizenship; neither of these can be simply granted but are negotiated in the process of claims being made. There is a need to ensure that **civic education courses** are provided which pay attention to issues around the provision of public welfare services.

The Challenge for Staff and Trade Unions

Public service workers and their trade unions have been facing challenging times and will continue to do so over the next decade. They have suffered a crisis of identity and purpose, accused of failing to adapt to changing needs and conditions and to deliver a sufficiently high quality of service. Their initial reaction was often to take a defensive stance, resisting change or avoiding engagement with new concepts and methods. However trade unions and public employees are now following a bolder, more proactive strategy, recognising the need for public services to adapt in order to remain relevant and sustainable. They see the need to be involved in the debate on key questions such as the role and responsibilities of public services, including those in the welfare area; the quality of their management; the role of the private and not-for-profit sectors; how to ensure efficiency, effectiveness and democratic control, as well as issues of pay and working conditions.

Evidence from the Foundation's research points to the need for change programmes in the public welfare services to take a **more dynamic view of the roles and responsibilities of staff**. This applies particularly to front line staff, who are the main interface between the service organisation and its users and who play a crucial role in any reform to improve the effectiveness and quality of service provision. In particular the research points to the following as meriting greater attention:-

1.   Public service staff should be **involved** more actively at all stages of reform programmes from the earliest phase of design and planning through to the monitoring, review and assessment of the innovations. The commitment and involvement of staff are essential if public welfare services are to meet current and future needs especially in the context of static or reduced resources. Managers need to recognise the value of this staff resource and the potential for improving services by learning from staff experiences and ideas.

2.   Staff at all levels must have access to adequate and appropriate **training**, both initially and in the course of their careers so as to:

-       develop skills and qualifications, including in relation to the introduction of information and other technology;

-       increase motivation, commitment and an understanding of new procedures, roles, standards and goals;

-       develop new ways of working with users and a better understanding of the causes and processes of poverty and exclusion;

- take on greater responsibility and to stimulate initiative and creativity;
- develop communication and negotiating skills;
- handle new tasks such as advice and counselling activities, and increased discretionary powers in meeting individual users' needs;
- promote cultural change in service organisations and generate changes in mentality and habits.

3.   There is need to pay greater attention to **working conditions issues** such as pay, grading structures, recruitment and promotion practices, job content, working methods and work environment. This can lead to a more motivated and productive workforce without necessarily adding to costs. The links between improvements in working conditions and improvements in service to users need to be clarified and stressed. A reform or innovation programme provides the opportunity to achieve multiple goals in several areas. More emphasis on bottom-up approaches building on the ideas from front line staff and from users can assist this process.

4.   Recognition should be given to the impact of change on, and the varying interests of, **different groups of staff** (professionals, clerical, administrative and manual). Open procedures, communication and negotiation can play important roles in balancing and understanding their different concerns.

5.   Moves to decentralise, co-ordinate and integrate different services provide new challenges to staff, who may be more likely to work in **multi-disciplinary teams** and to be involved in more complex information flows. Support must be given to facilitate these new working methods.

6.   The **time factor** plays an important role in change programmes. Staff will need sufficient time to adjust to change. Implementation plans need to be flexible but should avoid excessive delays. Continuity and strength of support must be evident from the top.

7.   **Recognition and support** should be available to staff taking on greater responsibility and stressful discretionary decisions. The gendered nature of many public service bureaucracies, traditionally run on hierarchical and patriarchal principles, needs to be recognised. There is a general tendency to underestimate or disregard the needs and views of **women** who frequently occupy the lower paid and front line jobs.

In relation to the role of **trade unions,** evidence points to a need to advocate positive change in public services which responds to genuine public concerns and which can win public support. Unions have a particular role to play in promoting proposals to improve service quality, improvements in working conditions and work environment and the involvement of staff in all stages of the change process.

There is a role here for national and workplace **collective agreements** which can set out public service objectives (quality, equity, democratic control) as well as pay, job design and working conditions, training and participation structures (such as the agreements in UK local government made in 1994). In the Foundation's case studies the role of unions at the local level appears in general to be weakly developed. There is increasing activity at European level with efforts to develop **social dialogue** in this area as well as a **European Charter for Public Services** and promotion of the contribution of public services to the fight against unemployment and social exclusion.

It would be in the interests of staff and trade unions to explore and encourage **new forms of management theory and practice** which would endorse the ethical values and quality of public services. It is as frustrating for employees as for service users if a service is poorly led and managed. Public service unions and their leaders should play a stronger role in negotiating at all levels the introduction, implementation and assessment of change and assisting in sending out the right signals to the staff they represent.

Implications for Managers and Policy Makers

Public welfare services have been affected in all the countries covered by this report by broader programmes of reform and modernisation in public administration and services. Much of the impetus for change has been external rather than internal, arising from political, economic, social and technological pressures which have forced the pace and pattern of change. However increasingly in many Member States, internal management is actively promoting, and committed to improving, both administrative effectiveness and quality of service. A strong top down approach to change, co-ordinated and inspired from the highest political levels is sometimes apparent. Elsewhere the role of local government has been crucial in conducting and funding change. This is strongly influenced by the different national systems and traditions in the public sector. The following guidelines for action at management and policy levels are put forward for consideration.

1.   **Political support** has been shown to be crucial to the success of change programmes providing inspiration, leadership and resources. There are dangers of reliance on single key individuals in the longer term but they can often provide important initial impetus for change. Putting change programmes and initiatives clearly in the political arena can also be important for users who can signal their views in common with other citizens at elections or in general contacts with politicians at the appropriate levels. Politicians should also be involved in the assessments of experiments and programmes and can provide support for the transfer of good practice.

2.   The significance of good **leadership** in instigating and sustaining change is very evident from the Foundation's research, together with the creation of **open organisational cultures** which encourage managers at different levels, staff and often users to experiment and learn by experience in the context of structured support from the top.

3.   New approaches will also require appropriate **management training** and the building of different competences. Policies of decentralisation, co-ordinated and

integrated service provision, staff and user involvement will have significant effects on the different levels of management. Issues of **power** and **changes of roles** are central to the reform process and will require new types of leadership, a willingness to develop shared goals and plans and a problem solving approach, often on a team basis, which emphasises opportunities and is clear about problems.

4. Particular attention will need to be paid to the production and transfer of **information** to staff, users and the public in general. This will form part of the necessary **technical and methodological support** for the change process but is also crucial in developing essential **monitoring, evaluation and review** procedures. There is a need here for more **research** to determine the practical impacts of the large number of experiments taking place. This work can also provide feedback to further improve services and develop future priorities. This assessment should also take account of the perspectives of the different stakeholders-users, staff and managers and be available to all citizens. **Transfer** and **diffusion** of good practice is also dependent on this process. It is suggested that the establishment of a central office at national level could assist in filling the current lack of effective evaluation and dissemination.

5. There is insufficient attention paid to issues of **equity** and **equal opportunities** in reform programmes, issues which are perhaps of particular significance in the public welfare area. Equality strategies, in their widest sense encompassing aspects of gender, race, age and sexual orientation, should form an integral part of change programmes to improve public services. This is particularly important if they are to make an impact on processes of **social exclusion**. Any failure to take account of the fact that users are not a homogenous group, even within one target group, is likely to disadvantage the most vulnerable. They are more likely to depend on public services, less likely to play an active involved role and less likely as citizens to bring influence to the political arena. This is little exploration of whether the same treatment for all users is in fact equal treatment. There is also the issue of

equal opportunities in employment practices, in access to training and career development and the need to develop the full potential of all public service staff.

6. There is a need for both **institutional reform** and for the development of **new approaches and structures,** examples of which are given earlier in this report. These can be complementary and provide greater flexibility in the face of rapid and often unpredictable economic and social change. In both cases however there is a requirement for adequate resources and for continuity of support if the changes are to bear fruit. National and local authorities can assist this process by the provision of incentive and pilot scheme funding for innovative projects and the nurturing of community based projects.

7. The identification and dissemination of techniques to **strengthen local democracy** as a means of securing improved accountability and consumer representation in public welfare services should be pursued as should other methods to support and develop the capacity of users and citizens to act as working partners with providers and policy makers.

The Contribution of the European Union

At European Union level the different institutions have been taking an increasing interest in public services from a number of different perspectives. The **Economic and Social Committee** in an Own Initiative Opinion in 1993, emphasised that an effective public service is a vital requirement to strengthen economic and social cohesion. The Committee highlighted, in particular the need for better staff training, promotion of innovation and exchange of experience, and regular joint consultation between public authorities, trade unions and consumer organisation. It identified also a number of areas where it felt the European Commission could play a role in stimulating training and trans-national exchange and in developing reference frameworks.

Up to now, action in relation to public services at European Union level has been concerned primarily with the application of Single Market and Treaty rules in relation to competition, mainly in the area of public utilities. However, the extension of welfare pluralism and an increased role for the private sector in health and social services as well as the strengthening of consumer protection policy under the Maastricht Treaty, provide a basis for increased competence and action at EU level.

In 1994 the Consumer Policy Service of the **European Commission** launched a major study on the public services in the Member States so as to analyze the different legal forms and the specific rules concerning users. It is also examining the development of Citizen's Charters and similar instruments and is seeking to develop a European Charter for consumers/citizens who use public services. Other key issues being examined are the provision of information, problems of access, redress/complaints procedures and the participation and representation of consumers/users. The Commission services have also undertaken research to examine questions of improving access to public services by disadvantaged users and the potential for a citizen's passport to services as a means of combatting social exclusion and poverty.

Chapter 2 of this report pointed to the general developments at EU level which have implications for the overall policy environment in this area. The recent Medium-Term Social Action Programme will be an important framework within which further developments relevant to the subject matter of this report can take place.

The fight against social exclusion requires efficient public services, which are also indispensable to ensure another key goal of the Union the ensuring of equal opportunities and equal treatment. The European Union has the potential to contribute to improvements in public services, including those in the welfare area in the following ways:

-       financial and technical support for the modernisation and reform of public services as part of the process of EU integration with the use of EU Structural Instruments;

- support for increased training of staff and management in the provision of quality, consumer-responsive services, for example through the European Social Fund;

- support for the transfer and exchange of knowledge, expertise and staff to facilitate dissemination and good practice;

- creation and analysis of relevant data, for example within the context of the Targeted Socio-Economic Research Programme (Activity 1.VII of the 4th Framework Research Programme 1994-1998);

- support for the development of social dialogue in the area of public services (problems in identifying an agreed employers' platform has caused some delay in this area);

- consideration of a European level forum which could provide a structure specifically for the representation and consultation of consumers of public services;

- the development of policies to strengthen the protection of consumers of public services, including policies on information, consultation, access and redress;

- strengthen support for networking between users' groups at local, national and European level, which is already developing to a certain extent through specialised social action programmes such as those for the disabled, older people and women;

- encourage and support more integrated, holistic and multidimensional responses by public welfare services to social and economic exclusion as recommended by the EU's Poverty 3 Programme;

- provide resources for greater experimentation and for demonstration projects to enable public welfare services to respond to growing problems of exclusion and poverty, especially in areas where traditionally these services are underdeveloped and bureaucratic in approach;

- include the issue of the improvement of the quality and effectiveness of public welfare services in all relevant social action programmes at EU level.

It is hoped that this report and the research from which it is drawn can act as a catalyst to stimulate debate and action on these issues. It is clear from the interest already expressed at national and international levels, and from many of the key actors, in the work of the Foundation in this area that this subject is of increasing concern. Significant international meetings have already been held over the past year to exchange experience and identify good practice (OECD, EPSC/ETUC). It is the Foundation's intention, together with the services of the European Commission to hold a European conference to stimulate debate on the role of public welfare services in the fight against social exclusion in the course of 1995. However, this research has highlighted the role and contribution of a great range of agencies, public bodies, and interest groups across the Member States. The proposals put forward in these conclusions will, it is hoped, act to fuel debate and to stimulate further action at the appropriate levels.

APPENDIX 1   GLOSSARY OF TERMS EMPLOYED

Public Welfare Services: those services provided by governments (central, regional and local) for social protection of their populations 'in the sense of the State assuming ultimate responsibility for the health and welfare of its citizens'.

Citizen: a status that derives from full legal membership of a collectivity, which confers certain rights and obligations. The rights include the exercise of choice through participation in political processes. Citizenship also involves entitlements to public goods and services on collectively agreed terms.

Users: individuals in their capacity as recipients of public welfare services. The ultimate beneficiaries of services may not be direct users of them; and users of certain services may not have chosen to receive them. Citizens who are not users have a broader interest in the cost and efficiency of these services. The term 'clients' is sometimes employed in a similar sense.

Consumers: individuals (both citizens and non-citizens) who obtain services through the market or from systems operated on market principles. These may be provided either by the state or through private or 'third sector' organisations. Choice and redress are secured by the operation of market mechanisms or procedures based upon them. The term 'customers' is sometimes used in the same sense; but normally implies a cash exchange for goods or services.

Empowerment: a term used to describe the situation in which power is transferred from the provider to the consumer, so that the latter enjoys control over future transactions. Often employed rhetorically but rarely encountered in practice (and therefore sometimes misleading).

Social Exclusion: the process through which individuals or groups are wholly or partially excluded from full participation in the society within which they live. Can be caused either by failure to secure employment (exclusion from the labour market) or by limited access to benefits or social services. This may be related to absence of full citizen rights (see above).

Social Dumping: the phenomenon by which certain national governments limit either the level of benefits or access to social protection, in an attempt to lower the cost of labour and encourage employers to invest or locate in their country.

APPENDIX 2 Case Studies in Depth: Seven examples of key issues in action

Apart from providing an analysis of the more significant outcomes from the case studies, we believe that it is helpful to provide a description in greater depth of some examples of the case studies which appear to us to have thrown up issues of particular importance, which need to be seen in the context of specific local circumstances. In this way the mixed dynamics and characteristics of changes and the interplay between various factors can also be illustrated.

1.   Kapis (Day care for elderly), Greece

This is a case of a policy innovation at national level, first conceived and introduced as a result of the initiative of an individual civil servant, then taken up through its congruence with national political agendas and adopted and promoted at local level, through the political system. The study covers the programme both at national level and in one specific locality (Nea Ionia).

The programme took a considerable while to establish itself, passing through a sequence of advocacy, acceptance, limited experiment (through the voluntary sector) to widespread adoption. The context is of a system of social welfare that is barely developed in any detail and lacks solid base in a professional group. Local government (which eventually assumed responsibility for the programme) lacked expertise both in the welfare field and generally (there is a tradition of very narrow range of functions and highly bureaucratised delivery of services).

Although the initial experimental Kapis were not formally evaluated, the programme was consistent with the incoming Socialist government's policies in two areas: decentralisation of more responsibility to local government and deinstitutionalisation of care. Once adopted and resourced, Kapis also fitted local agenda. In the specific case study area, the programme was personally adopted by the local mayor, who promoted it energetically. The future of the scheme is now less certain, partly because of a change of funding arrangements which means that the project is now funded out of the general grant to local authorities rather than through a specific one (which has brought up the question of how far Kapis are appropriate as a high priority at a time of increased pressure on spending).

A striking feature of the project is the relatively high priority assigned to users. They are involved in planning the service, through membership of the Kapis local board of management (chaired by the Mayor). They also have considerable informal influence on the content of the services provided at the Kapis, which in the Nea Ionia case have increasingly tended to stress leisure facilities and informal 'club' arrangements. (In terms of categories set out earlier, users are probably best conceived of as 'junior partners': there is a comment that their expectations are not high and the new services are not seen as a right).

The content of the Nea Ionia Kapis activities does not necessarily fit with staff priorities. Another important feature of the scheme is the lack of any managerial 'core': the staff consists of specialists from a range of social service and medical disciplines; residual administrative tasks have been delegated to the local authority and are performed at 'arms length'. The staff group see their role as reasserting the original values of the Kapi experiment and also protecting their own position at a time of cutbacks (Greek bureaucratic rules mean that their position is probably secure).

Thus, voice in the Greek case is exercised largely by the staff; although the role of local government means that the system is accountable to citizens as voters, subject to the constraints of limited resources as well as to users. Choice can be exercised by users within the scope of the Kapi; but no alternative facilities exist outside it. Access is one of the major gains; services which were either not available or very difficult or expensive to reach are now accessible to Kapi members. Energetic promotion of the concept by the Socialists during their period in power means that there are now 65,000 users of this service; however, this falls far short of the potential numbers.

2.   Wiltshire Community Care User Involvement Network (WCCUIN), United Kingdom

This initiative, which was launched in 1991, has had success in developing user led user involvement. It is a network of service users, advocates and carers who work with staff from community care services including health, social service, voluntary and private agencies to design and develop services for disabled and older people in the County of Wiltshire.

The impetus for this development came partly from a growing disability movement seeking to empower its members, but it can also be traced to changes in national policy regarding the provision of services to older people, disabled people, people with learning disabilities and people with mental health problems. These changes, initiated in the late 1980s were directed at radically changing the role of local authority Social Service Departments in Britain. From being the main providers of formal care and services for adults needing care in the community Social Service Departments have been given a remit by government to assess need in this area, and co-ordinate the delivery of care purchased from a mix of statutory, voluntary and private organisations. This is to be the latest means of achieving the long-term policy goal of de-institutionalisation and a consequential shift in responsibility from health to social care.

As part of these changes Social Service Departments were required by government to develop, through consultation, a Community Care Plan for their locality. In 1991 in Wiltshire this consultation process initially involved just four service users. These users decided that they wanted to establish a user network in the County in order to prevent the marginalisation of users in influencing the changing community care services. The aims of the network were to address the isolation of service users and to establish an organisation which through user-leadership promoted the involvement and empowerment of service users in a changing service environment.

By 1993 the network had extended its membership to 260 individuals and contact with 120 user groups. It organises itself through an elected planning group of 16 members, 12 of whom are service users who meet monthly. The Network uses a newsletter, the telephone and regular membership meetings on current issues and developments to develop its role. It supports a range of groups and individual activities and initiatives with both local and national service and carer organisations. Its terms of reference are to:

*   raise awareness of issues of, and opportunities for, user involvement in community care provision
*   promote user involvement and disseminate examples of good practice of user involvement in community care provision in the voluntary, statutory and private sectors
*   act as a Wiltshire network for policy and planning issues related to service user involvement in Community Care.

This initiative promotes the view that service users of community care services are active agents in respect to the management of their own lives. It challenges longstanding professional notions of passive service recipients with needs that require professional assessment and servicing. In this work it has drawn sustenance and contributed to a national climate in which there are a growing number of organisations of people with disabilities who have developed a critique of professional practice and campaigned for the introduction of anti-discriminatory legislation for disabled people. While the majority of service users are women, the Network has not explicitly addressed some of the gendered assumptions of service purchasers and providers.

The Network was created and has been promoted by the energies and commitment of user members and their allies drawn from professional workers and carers. It had been successful in securing funding from the local authority for its activities. The fact that the Director of the Social Services Department has been receptive to this development and has been identified as a "champion for change" has been an important factor in the success of this initiative.

The Network's commitment to building an empowering and participative organisation is reflected in the way it has worked from the outset to provide access, support and encouragement to individuals to meet together and, by speaking out about their experiences and needs, to advocate for themselves.

The Network has aimed to work with service staff in dialogue and through alliances. Thus it has challenged professional perceptions, attitudes and practices where these have had the effect of disempowering users. Workers and managers have experienced the difficulties of responding to a changing culture, and the responses have been mixed.

As we have noted, this change in culture and expectations was taking place at a time when radical changes to organisation of delivery of community care were part of national and local agendas. Resource constraint in the face of increasing demands from the client group was a feature of the daily lives of staff delivering services in all sectors. How this tension arising from rationing resources in the face of increased user involvement was being managed by predominantly female staff is an issue which deserves further scrutiny.

3.   Ballyfermot One-Stop Shop, Ireland

This is a case of a top-down initiative planned by a central government department as part of a wider range of new national policies on delivery of welfare services. The provision of a 'one stop' service in purpose-built premises for an area suffering from a combination of high unemployment, multiple social problems and a poor environment was part of an attempt to address problems of social exclusion more effectively. Its introduction had also been strongly advocated by local politicians and by residents, who had to contend with low quality, fragmented and inaccessible services.

The project is best seen as a thoroughgoing reform of an existing service - both in the sense of a structural change (grouping of previously separated provision) but also an attempt to achieve a qualitative change in the level of service delivered. In this process, the provision of better information, facilitated by the introduction of new technology, has played an important part, as has improvement in the style of service delivery, through staff training.

Users have not been actively involved in the process of reform. The change in their situation could be summed up as a move from client to customer status. It is clear from a brief, small scale study of user attitudes that a marked improvement in quality of provision and standard of service is perceived; and this is confirmed by the attitude of local community groups, who also appreciate the shift in staff attitudes towards greater acceptance of the rights of users.

The response of staff is mixed. The original decision to provide the new service has the support of the unions; and the quality of the premises and the level of technical support provided is seen as a clear gain. There has also been a good response to the training provided and the option of working nearer home, has been helpful for dual career female staff. However, some members of staff see their situation as having been affected by the very high levels of tension and stress involved in the content of work. Finally, the new form of provision in a single office is seen as having opened up new career opportunities for women members of staff (previously disadvantaged here).

In terms of outcomes, the issue of voice barely arises, although limited attempts to secure an assessment by users have taken place. Choice, too, is not relevant in a situation where most clients have no option to turn to but benefits (in effect, they are captives of the welfare system). However, better accessibility is a key gain, both in terms of geographical access and a more user-friendly style of service delivery, and is clearly seen as such by users (But what about the disabled or women with children? Apparently the interview room for the Community Welfare Officer is upstairs. There is also no systematic provision for reception). Finally, accountability is somewhat remote. There is a new regional system of delivery; but main accountability would be through the political system, and it appears that local politicians have been active in pressing for improved standards of service.

4.   **Tribunale per i Diritti del Malato (Patients' Rights Tribunals), Italy**

The Patients' Tribunals are unique among our case studies, in that they represent a nation-wide, largely grass-roots social movement, whose presence has spread rapidly since it began in 1980. The emergence of such movements would be unlikely, but for the convergence of several significant trends. Pre-eminent among these was the growing crisis of confidence in the Italian state and its processes of governance as well as its ability to deliver effective services. One reaction to this has been the seizure of the modernising vision and opportunities created by the "historic appointment with Europe". A new national health service, in which professionals retained a strong voice, but were joined by managers in a co-ordinated structure, is one example. It created its own reaction. This reaction was made possible by two developments: the growing citizen interest in reclaiming health and the decision-making around it; and the development of a "Democracy Federation" as an alternative, countervailing force to established political parties.

Patients' tribunals thus began with the collation of hundreds of complaints and the stirring of local self-help organisations sponsored by the Democratic Federation. The rapid localised spread of these initiatives during the 1980s led to action on a national front towards the end of the decade. This status was institutionalised at the beginning of the 90s through a legislative decree giving the tribunals formal rights of representation, as well as support for a national survey of patients' rights.

The activities of groups vary locally, but many of them encompass a range of action. The development of patients' charters and other service standards is one: more commonly, local agreements are negotiated and monitored, without their formal proclamation. The tribunals also mediate between users and professionals - including over the latter's rights to strike. Lobbying and advocacy may also occur, which may include action to support vulnerable minorities, such as the rights of women in labour, and the protection of elderly people from the impact of national policy proposals. Specific actions on behalf of women as carers concern such things as access for mothers of children in paediatric wards, and improvement in hospital food, so that female relatives are not forced to bring it daily. Speedier outpatient appointments have also benefitted women as patients and carers. Campaigns against closure of services have also been mounted. Here and elsewhere, use of the mass media has been an important weapon.

Additionally, the local tribunals may also become involved in training initiatives for professionals and, on occasion, have undertaken direct service provision, where alternative agencies could not be found (especially in primary care).

The tribunals make common cause with professionals as appropriate. At a collective level these may be protests against closure or pressure to develop new services. At an individual level many professional staff are members of their local tribunals, while it is estimated that 25,000 staff act as potential whistle-blowers when things go wrong. Such coalitions have developed over time, from initially conflictual relations. Over time, significant shifts in attitude have taken place among staff, both as regards the validity of a wider voice and the importance of user comfort, access and inter-personal relations, which would otherwise tend to be neglected in favour of technical and therapeutic concerns. Thus, the frames of reference and working practices of some professionals - especially nurses - have been modified. Such changes are likely to be reinforced by managerial quality initiatives.

In the context of current financial stringency, relations between tribunals and professionals may work in two directions: common cause to resist cuts and campaign for better services, speedier access and shorter queues; and also pressure on beleaguered staff not to jeopardise the comfort of patients. One route out of this dilemma is the current 'war on waste'.

Access to decision makers is also said to have improved over the years, both at local and national levels. Thus the tribunals have increasingly gained insider status as spokespeople for otherwise excluded interests. This has been particularly important as a counter to the trend to concentrate responsibility into the hands of managers, rather than representative committees. The space created by the decline of political parties is also important in this respect.

The movement is based largely on voluntary effort and so, to an extent, is its funding. On the other hand, local and national management fund certain activities and may provide accommodation and similar support.

Local variation and the limited availability of any evaluation prevents any judgement about the extent to which the presence and vitality of voluntary activity is linked to socio-economic or similar factors, so that no full assessment of who is included or excluded from this movement is possible. Certainly, some potentially excluded groups, such as people with mental health problems or learning disabilities have been incorporated or their interests taken up.

Equally, it is not entirely clear how far the movement is transferable, since it is not a project, but a "complex, articulated network of essentially autonomous groups and individuals", shaped by its local context and the broader national context which afforded the conditions of its creation. This should not detract however, from real gains in voice, accountability and the provision of accessible and acceptable services.

5.   The Amadora Office of the Lisbon Social Security Centre, Portugal

The dynamics for this initiative combine a national policy directive with a particularly energetic and facilitating local management style and a responsive staff group. In the mid 1980s the national government of Portugal launched a national public service initiative which aimed to increase service accessibility; optimise human resources; improve service management, and improve service delivery through the de-bureaucratisation of procedures. Within this programme the social security and social welfare services, which co-ordinate a mix of public and private services were given a remit to promote greater social justice, make better social provision and promote equal opportunity.

The Amadora Office was opened in 1988 but was adapted in 1990 to provide a complete range of social security and social welfare services for the municipality of Amadora. The female managers of the service and the mostly female staff group worked closely together to deliver an improved, personalised service to a group of service users who traditionally come from the most disadvantaged groups in the community and of whom 75% are women. This work was undertaken using the tools set by national government. What singled this service out was the friendly, personal service that managers and staff were able to deliver to service users from the local community.

No systematic service evaluation was built into this initiative and it was the research on which this study was based which provided the main means of assessing the impact of the change in service style on service users and staff. A survey of service users indicated that they valued the friendly reception they received from staff, the good physical environment of the office and the accessible information provided by the office about a range of available services. It was interesting to note that the researchers found that majority of service users were unused to being asked their opinions of this service and a number were unable to respond confidently to some of the questions they were asked.

Staff and managers of the services demonstrate a strong commitment and pride in the quality of the service they were creating for service users and the improvement they experienced in their working conditions and job satisfaction. New ideas about procedures and service style were evolving in a climate where staff felt valued and supported.

6.   Arche Rostock eV (The Rostock Ark), Germany

The Ark is a voluntary organisation, set up in 1991, providing employment through job creation schemes and, in doing so, building or renovating accommodation which affords housing and social facilities for disadvantaged minority groups.

The cross-cutting mix of social employment and social provision, and the unstable coalitions of quite diverse agencies and informal groups is typical of many earlier schemes in the Federal Republic. Indeed this diffusion to the new states is based upon the "Planning Workshop" in the twin city of Bremen and its successful adoption owes much to the enthusiasm and expertise of a Bremen academic.

The innovative element of the scheme is that many of its key actors are leading officials of the local authority, working voluntarily through this intermediary agency. This enables the Ark to act as an intermediary between the local authority and various grassroots initiatives, to operate flexibly and informally in ways not open to a public bureaucracy, to receive external funds and to benefit from the synergy of working at the interface between town planning, employment policy and social and youth services. In this way, too, it acts as a catalyst to service developments to be run for and by minority informal organisations, giving them access to networks, funds and an organisational infrastructure - and, eventually, accommodation which they would not otherwise enjoy. The organisation also benefits from high level political support.

The push factors making such radical actions possible relate to a rapidly declining local economy, with high unemployment and under-employment, heavy reliance of special employment measures, a growing reliance on social security, high outward migration, a low tax yield leading to extreme financial stringency, job cuts, and heavy reliance on Federal and State grants. High levels of social unrest accompanied these problems, with crises around attacks on asylum-seekers and the occupation of buildings precipitating action. In addition, the absence of formal intermediary bodies and informal networks forced the city authority to the fore, at the same time as pre-occupying some potentially key departments with the establishment of such organisations.

The pull factors came in the form of political support for radical and innovative action, the growing self-organisation of minorities, the example, expertise and continued guidance of the Bremen consultant and the dedication and enthusiasm of people forming the core of the implementation network they set up. The availability of job creation funds from the Federal Ministry of Employment and grants to finance training from the European Social Fund were also a crucial pre-requisite and a crucial determinant of the shape of the project. The crisis and the need for positive models of social re-integration and control provided the legitimacy for the project.

Ark's first enterprise was to offer employment to a group of punks occupying a building: they could renovate some alternative accommodation, receive training and a right to rent a flat in the re-furbished building. The self-help organisation they formed is a member of Ark, thus gaining a voice in its deliberations. Subsequently, Ark has been working with a self-help group of single parent students, re-furbishing housing which that group will subsequently manage. This arose from a successful bid for funds for experimental accommodation projects for single parents. Another building will act as a home base for various groups - including a parent and child initiative and a leisure centre to be run by and for disabled people. Further projects include a youth and cultural centre on a run-down estate (for which Ark also facilitates inter-agency planning), a kindergarten and a field centre for a school.

This progress has been achieved on the basis of fragile foundations. Lack of any core funding from the outset led to the overcommitment and subsequent withdrawal of the initial voluntary activists, when their official paid work for the local authority suffered. Subsequent volunteers have now been incorporated as paid staff, but most of the professionals involved as administrators, educational sociologists and so on are paid from the same temporary job creation funds as the young men doing the re-furbishment, so the growing professionalism of the project is at some risk. Training activities are contracted to a partner organisation and Ark has decided to stick to its knitting of building renovation, so that it needs other organisations and groups to help design and then run any social services which are made possible.

These fragile foundations were also to be seen in ad hoc management arrangements and a fluid set of relationships and personnel between governing body and working officers of the organisation. The management of the housing project for punks - the first project - remains to be determined, for example.

The reseachers suggest that user empowerment is neither particularly evident nor particularly useful as a criterion for judging the success of the employment elements of the project. In their view, the building workers (then numbering 140 people) are sent by the employment office and are in insufficient control of rather chaotic lifestyles to recognise and begin to meet their own needs, let alone become full partners. Of the 17 punks originally starting work on the first scheme, over half had been subsequently dismissed. Rather the quality of the training and the counselling about this and other aspects of their lives are the crucial determinants of the value they derive and even their continued access to their opportunity. Hence the need for professionalism and some security among core staff.

However, Ark does provide the necessary infrastructure to enable other self-help groups to gain access to physical, technical, financial, political and human resources, so that they will have something to self-manage. It is at this point that users can be empowered. They are all minority interest communities - which by definition entails the exclusion of other interests. In this respect it is significant that the only single parents to be helped will be students and while the indigenous young unemployed men, similar to those who burned down a hostel for asylum seekers, are targets for help, their victims are not.

In like vein, women gain largely by being beneficiaries of new services, rather than being employed to create them. This is equally true of disabled people. Thus the economic benefits and training go mostly to young men, despite higher rates of female unemployment. Perhaps ironically, most of those in the core posts - highly demanding, uncertain work with an emphasis on networking, flexibility and ad-hocery - are women.

A similar irony is that it was the lack of resources, the absence of elaborated, established, specialised and thus inflexible organisations - as well as territories to defend - which led to a local authority taking imaginative and adventurous action. Can similar lessons be learned by the wealthy, or must crisis and necessity precede invention?

7.   Hyldespjaeldet Social Network, Denmark

In this case, the initiative comes from the local level - a self-managed housing cooperative with executive power resting with the estate committee. For the purpose of this project, the residents chose to hand over authority to a small informal group ('the gang of four'), which took responsibility for developing a number of specific action schemes.

The proposal stemmed from the failure of earlier more formal schemes to address deep seated problems of social and economic deprivation on the estate, taking the highly visible form of a group of unemployed young people, heavily involved in drug and alcohol abuse. Resources for a new approach were obtained through an application to the research branch of the Ministry of Social Affairs; the project was presented as a self-help initiative resting on the ability of the community to generate constructive solutions to its main problems through networking which would release skills among the residents themselves.

Three specific schemes were generated in this way: one to address youth unemployment, one to support local patients at a psychiatric hospital and one to provide additional community facilities on the estate. These schemes were facilitated by a fulltime officer employed by the estate executive committee. The character of the project as a whole was highly experimental and initially it had only very limited funding, relying heavily on the resident networks to deliver. However, as the project progressed it proved possible to 'shake loose' more financial resources from various special funds managed by public agencies.

The individual schemes had a variety of outcomes. The young unemployed were involved in estate maintenance and repair and given some additional training; the scheme succeeded in containing the public order problem on the estate but was less successful in enabling those who completed the schemes to move successfully into the job market. The scheme for setting up a network to help psychiatric patients foundered on adverse press publicity. And the 'culture cafe' that was opened, though initially successfully in attracting support from residents and supporting a fulltime member of staff, eventually had to be reorganised on a less ambitious basis. Criteria of success evidently differed as between residents, who saw the outcomes in terms of visible benefits for the estate and the local authority, who were quite reserved about the project as a whole and its limited wider impact (schemes didn't get enough people off the dole).

Users were clearly managers in this case. This brought tensions as well as rewards. The 'gang of four', the legitimacy of whose authority was not always clear, fell out with fellow residents about the appointment of the successor to the fulltime worker - their wish to appoint a resident who was one of their own associates was not popular. Users were also co-producers, in the sense that the networks delivered a good deal of unpaid work in support of the individual initiatives; the expectation was that this involvement would also entitle residents to share in defining or modifying objectives. The local authority's rather remote attitude meant that there was no countervailing force setting alternative objectives.

The situation of the staff was equivocal. The insecurity of working conditions and the closeness to the employers (in the shape of the local community) were balanced by close involvement in an experiment with some exciting outcomes.

In terms of outcome measures, voice was freely exercised in the internal debates which also gave the organisers and participants a substantial degree of choice. Access appears to have been no problem within the local community; but their representatives had very considerable difficulty in securing access to the local authority and gaining their support. Accountability, finally, was clearly present in the highly democratic local structures - and control was exercised in the case of the episode of the staff appointment.

APPENDIX 3 **NATIONAL REPORTS AVAILABLE FROM THE EUROPEAN FOUNDATION FOR THE IMPROVEMENT OF LIVING AND WORKING CONDITIONS ON WHICH THIS CONSOLIDATED REPORT IS BASED**

1.   Castello-Branco, Maria Jose (1994) Consumer-Oriented Action in Public Services in Portugal. Estudos e Projectos, Lisbon. EFILWC, WP/94/28/PT

2.   Christofferson, Henrik and Hansen, Eigil Boll (1994) The Development of the Consumer Orientation in the Public Services in Denmark. AFK, Copenhagen. EFILWC, WP/94/25/EN,DA.

3.   D'Andrea, Luciano and Cioli, Patrizia (1994) Consumer-Oriented Action in the Public Services - General analysis and case studies for Italy. CERFE, Rome. EFILWC, WP/94/27/EN,IT.

4.   Hoggett, Paul (1994) Consumer-Oriented Action in the Public Services, National Report for the United Kingdom. University of Bristol, School for Advanced Urban Studies, Bristol. EFILWC, WP/94/23/EN

5.   Jani-Le Bris, Hannelore and Luquet, Valerie (1994) Consumer-Oriented Action in the Public Services in France. CLEIRPPA, Paris. EFILWC, WP/../../EN,FR.

6.   Kern, Kristine, Lang, Andrea, Wegrich, Kai and Wollmann, Hellmut (1994) Consumer-Oriented Action in the Public Services - German Case Studies. Free University of Berlin. EFILWC, WP/94/26/EN,DE.

7.   Leigh-Doyle, Sue and Mulvihill, Ray (1994) Consumer-Oriented Action in Public Services in Ireland. Leigh-Doyle and Associates, Dublin. EFILWC, WP/94/24/EN.

8.   Varelidis, Nikos (1994) Consumer-oriented Action in Public Services, National Report for Greece. PRISMA - Centre for Development Studies, Athens. EFILWC, WP/95/36/EN.

A progress report on the first phase of the project is also available:
Consumer-Oriented Action in the Public Services: overview and progress report EFILWC, WP/94/01/EN.

RESEARCH ORGANISATIONS

AKF
Institute of Local Government Studies
Nyropsgade 37
DK-1602 Copenhagen V
Denmark

School for Advanced Urban Studies
University of Bristol
Rodney Lodge
Grange Road
Bristol BS8 4EA
United Kingdom.

PRISMA - Centre for Development Studies
17 Empedokleous Street
GR-11635 Athens
Greece

CLEIRPPA - Centre de Liaison,
d'Etude, d'Information et de Recherche
sur les Problemes des Personnes Agées
15, Rue Chateaubriand
F-75008 Paris
France

Leigh Doyle and Associates
73 Seabury
Sydney Parade Avenue
IRL-Dublin 4
Ireland

Institut für Politikwissenschaft
Humboldt Universität
Ziegelstraße 13c
D-1086 Berlin
Germany

Centro di Ricerca e
Documentazione Febbraio '74 (CERFE)
Via Flaminia 160
I-00196 Rome
Italy

Centro Estudos Direito Europeu
Instituto Superior Economis e Gestão
R. Miguel Lupi, 20
P-1200 Lisbon
Portugal

BIBLIOGRAPHY

Arnstein, S (1971) A Ladder of Citizen Participation. **Journal of The Royal Town Planning Institute. Vol 57,** No 4, pp176-182.

Baine, S, Benington, J and Russell, S (1992) **Changing Europe.** (London, NCVO).

Beresford, P and Croft, S (1993) **Citizen Participation.** (London, Macmillan).

Cecchini, P (1988) **The European Challenge, 1992.** (Aldershot, Wildwood House).

Danish National Institute of Social Research (1992) **Social Europe.** (Copenhagen, DNSIR).

Ditch, J (1993) 'The European Community: A Developing Social Dimension?' **Benefits, January/February No 6,** pp2-5.

ECOSOC (1993) Opinion on Future of Public Sector in Europe (Own-initiative Opinion 93/C 304/08).

Economist (1994) 'Europe and the Underclass; the slippery slope' (30.7).

Esping-Andersen, G (1990) **The Three Worlds of Welfare Capitalism.** Cambridge: Polity Press

European Commission (1993a) **Green Paper - European Social Policy: options for the Union.** (Luxembourg, EC).

European Commission (1993b) **Growth, Competitiveness and Employment.** (Luxembourg, EC).

European Commission (1994a) **White Paper - European Social Policy: a way forward for the Union.** (Luxembourg, EC).

European Commission (1994b) **White Paper, Part B - European Social Policy: a way forward for the Union.** Com (1994) 333.

European Commission (1994) **Report on Social Protection.** (Luxembourg, EC).

European Commission (1995) **Medium Term Social Action Programme 1995-1997,** Communication from the Commission to the Council and the European Parliament and to the Economic and Social Committee and the Committee of the Regions, Brussels.

European Foundation for the Improvement of Living and Working Conditions (1987) **Providing Information About Urban Services.** (Luxembourg, EC).

European Foundation for the Improvement of Living and Working Conditions (1990) **Public Services: Working for the Consumer**. (Luxembourg, EC).

European Foundation for the Improvement of Living and Working Conditions (1992) **Out of the Shadows** (Luxembourg, EC).

European Foundation for the Improvement of Living and Working Conditions (1994) **New Forms of Work: The Gender Dimension** (WP/94/55/EN).

European Foundation for the Improvement of Living and Working Conditions (1994) **Bridging the Gulf** (Luxembourg, EC).

European Public Services Committee (1994) **Public Services for the People of Europe. Common Agenda for Concerted and Joint Action**, Brussels.

Gaster, L and Taylor, M (1993) **Learning from Consumers and Citizens.** (Luton, Local Government Management Board).

Hantrais, L (1994) 'Comparing family policy in Britain, France and Germany' **Journal of Social Policy, 23,** 2, pp135-160.

Kleinman, M and Piachaud, D (1993) 'European Social Policy: conceptions and choices' **Journal of European Social Policy, 3,** 1, pp1-20.

The National Economic and Social Forum (1995) **Quality Delivery of Social Services**, Forum Report No. 6, Dublin.

OECD (1994) **Service Quality Initiatives in OECD Member Countries** (PUMA/PAC (94) 13).

Rhodes, R (1991) 'The New Public Management' **Public Administration Vol 69,** No 1, p. 1).

Smith, S R and Lipsky, M (1993) **Non-Profits for Hire: The Welfare State in the Age of Contracting.** Harvard UP.

United Kingdom Government (1991) **Citizen's Charter.** (London, HMSO).

United Kingdom Government (1994) **Competitveness and Employment: The UK Approach.** (London, HM Treasury and Department of Employment).

United Nations (1988) **World Population Prospects.** (New York, UN).

European Foundation for the Improvement of Living and Working Conditions

Public Welfare Services and Social Exclusion –
The development of consumer-oriented initiatives in the European Union

Luxembourg: Office for Official Publications of the European Communities

1995 – 164 pp. – 16 cm x 23.4 cm

ISBN 92-827-4907-X

Price (excluding VAT) in Luxembourg: ECU 18.50